SETTING UP YOUR OWN PREPAID PLAN

A Do-It-Yourself Guide

Dale E. Wagman, DDS

PennWell Publishing Company
1421 South Sheridan/ P.O. Box 1260
Tulsa, Oklahoma 74101

Library of Congress Cataloging-in-Publication Data

Wagman, Dale E.
Setting up your own prepaid plan: a do-it-yourself guide/ Dale E. Wagman
p. cm.
Includes index.
ISBN 0-87814-340-8
1. Dental economics — United States. 2. Dentistry — Practice — United States. 3. Insurance, Dental — United States. 4. Capitalism — United States. 5. Free Enterprise. I. Title.
RK58.5.W34 1989
368.3,823,0068 — dc19
89-30885
CIP

Printed in the United States of America

1 2 3 4 5 93 92 91 90 89

Table of Contents

SECTION IV
Topics Relevant to Capitation and PPO-Model Plans

APPENDICES

Preface

Throughout this country, many dentists watch as circumstances beyond their control gradually weaken their command of their own profession. They are besieged by countless plans, programs, and networks tugging at the purse strings of the industry, ultimately diluting the flow of cash to those professionals on the front lines who make it all work. Many have sought to regain some of that control and some of those dollars by starting programs and plans of their own. They watch as potential clients are lured away from their practices by lower costs. Many wonder how they can develop plans and programs of their own to win those clients back and prevent the loss of others as time goes on. The question *how* echoes and reverberates in their heads.

This book attempts to answer that question and to provide direction to front-line providers who have considered creating a dental plan intended to attract patients and keep them, and accomplish this goal in the easiest and most cost-efficient manner. It begins by describing what is currently available and defining the types of programs best-suited for provider development and operation. It then inspects the capitation plan, one of the most common of the new breed of financial mechanisms in health care and the type most often considered first by newcomers to the industry. Finally it outlines a relatively risk-free simplified plan which can be attempted by a practitioner or entrepreneur at any level.

Let me say at the outset that I realize that this book probably contains much more material than most providers will want to deal with. For those of you who are not interested in the complexities of setting up a capitation plan, I would suggest moving on to Section III, which deals with discount PPO plans, after reading the general overview in Section I.

Without question, this book is intended to dissuade some providers from entering into endeavors which would only waste their time, money, and energies. At the same time, it is intended to show others how a grass-roots movement could eventually restore control of an industry which works best by old-fashioned, fee-for-service, you-get-what-you-pay-for, free competition.

It is unfortunate that what appear to be simple ends should require such complicated means.

SECTION I

The Rationale for Prepaid Dental Programs

Chapter 1 Changing Attitudes

Your work load is as full as it could possibly be. You have no holes in your schedule. You are making all the money you could ever need. You look in your crystal ball and see this trend continuing indefinitely. If this is where you are, then don't bother reading this book. You are in the fortunate position of not needing prepaid dental plans in any form.

On the other hand, do you have a few holes in your schedule, or your associate's schedule, or are you thinking about opening a satellite office but are afraid you may not be able to attract enough patients? Is your view of the future clouded by the reality of a changing market for health care services? Are you smart enough to realize that the old manner in which dentists earned their money is going the way of the pterodactyl? Then use this book to familiarize yourself with the new trends in prepaid dentistry and develop a sense of how you can incorporate this concept into your daily practice.

A very long time ago, things were simple. People waited until they had "a little quickiness in a jaw tooth" or "needed an eye tooth floated" before they went to the dentist. He would take care of the problem and the patients would then do a strange thing: they would pay the dentist on the spot. Then, in 1954, attitudes changed—the patient's attitude, not the dentist's —and it's the attitude of the consumer that ultimately rules the behavior of providers, whether they are steel manufacturers, dentists, or hotdog vendors.

The first inklings of change occurred when one group of consumers, the International Longshoremen's and Warehousemen's Union (Pacific Maritime Association), decided they were working too hard and needed more money for their labors, not in itself a unique attitude change. They went on strike against the entire West Coast shipping industry. The shipping industry could not afford to pay all of the extra dollars the workers wanted, but through a slight attitude change of its own, the industry agreed to pay dental benefits for the workers instead of actual dollars. The union then made arrangements with the dental societies of the states of Washington, Oregon, and California to set up plans for implementation of the new program. Thus, the first Dental Service Corporation or Delta Plan was born. Not that other private insurance companies hadn't considered the idea, but no studies had been done to determine whether or not dental insurance could be underwritten. The new plan opened the door for a flood of indemnifying dental programs that would change the face of the entire industry, and elevate the science of dentistry to a new level.

Can you believe the dentists actually resisted the idea at first? Evidence can still be seen today in many of the ads for dentists in the yellow pages: "Most dental insurance plans accepted," as if there were still a dentist around who did not want to get paid by an insurance company.

Eventually the attitudes of dentists corrected for the new course and most profited handsomely. Profited for a while, that is, until the consumer dictated the next change by complaining to their congressmen that the cost of dentistry was too high. Actually, there are those who believe that in light of the beating insurance companies took once the ball got rolling, the next change was prompted by strong lobbying of third party insurers. Nonetheless, in an effort to curb rising costs in the dental segment, the federal government in cooperation with the state governments, launched many programs intended to increase the numbers of new dentists, diluting the provider base, increasing competition, and thereby lowering the overall cost of services. It was the old supply and demand shell game. The insurance companies stood behind the counter in silk shirts and black arm bands. They manipulated the shells, which were the numbers of practitioners and the regulations. The dentists stood around with their hands in their pockets trying to keep an eye on the elusive pea—this month's rent. The ploy worked well; just ask anyone trying to make it during the late '70s or early '80s. Practitioners who had been very successful for years were finding it difficult to make payroll, and some even went out of business. The competition was so strong that nobody did very well. This abundance of hungry doctors opened the doors for a new phenomenon—a new attitude change. Enter the entrepreneur!

The Birth of Capitation Plans

Businessmen noticed this pool of dental talent and the tremendous number of dollars that are spent each year on dental services. It was too much for them to stand. They reasoned that if they were to economize, share space, market, and manage an industry which was notorious for primitive managerial expertise, they could divert some of those dollars into their own pockets. New dental offices opened everywhere, inside shopping malls and over the 25-cent car wash, all made possible by the abundance of young doctors to staff them.

One thing leads to another, and one day an innovative entrepreneur sees all the new dental chairs sitting idle and decides the next game will be to get a portion of the bucks before they ever get to the patient/doctor interface. Talk about the stage being set! The insurance companies raised their prices in an effort to increase their corporate margins in a market where claims had increased dramatically. The employers, who for the most part had been hit hard by the ravages of a changing economy, looked at the increased premiums and swallowed hard. Individuals who had to share in premiums and then cough up a share of the cost directly to the dentist downright choked! And at the same time, there was a tremendous potential for delivery of services just waiting to be tapped. All the businessman had to do was to get the two sides together—unhappy consumers on one side, and on the other, dentists floundering like beached whales with useless advertising campaigns directed at those who are not inclined to come to the dentist anyway. A person could get rich on what spilled over when these two collided. Hello, capitation plans. Hello to a whole new series of attitude changes.

Losing money

The first major thing one has to accept about these new changes is that on the whole, you are going to lose money! While we're not talking about taking money out of your piggy bank and throwing it in the wood burner, we are talking about losing potential money. We're talking about losing some of the difference between what it actually costs you to perform a service, and what you would be paid on a strict fee-for-service basis. We're talking about losing some of your profit margin. Unfortunately, there is no other way. The consumer has spoken!

Let's say you charge $100 for a gold crown. The lab gets $15, $35 goes to your staff, and $30 goes for all the other bills around the office. And if all your ducks are properly lined up, you may get to take home $20. That is assuming the patient is willing to have the service in the first place. If not, you pay $65 to the staff and other creditors, and take home nothing. The worst business person in the world knows that won't work for long. Now, along comes a man selling prepaid dental plans. He is looking for a provider in your area and says, "I have a patient here who is willing to pay $82 for a crown. Are you willing to sell it to him?"

Pull out the calculator. Do the math real fast. "Let's see, lab $15, staff $35, rent, lights, everyone else gets paid and that leaves $2 for me. Well that's better than nothing. God knows I've got the time. I'll do it!"

This example may seem extreme, but the point is valid. The buzz word from the payer's side of the spectrum is "cost containment." It doesn't really matter what type of plan it is—capitation, PPO, IPA, or HMO. The money has to come from somewhere. The consumer has chosen that it come from the dentist. If you find that disgusting, or simply intolerable, your options are to leave the profession, accept your practice the way it is now, or change your attitude.

Let's look a little more closely at the example. The dentist, through co-pays and/or shares of the premium paid by capitation reimbursements, or kick-backs, or whatever, took in $82. But, the patient actually paid a total of $92 for the service. It was a good deal for him, since he saved $8. What happened to the $10? It went to someone else! The dentist took the risk of providing an often unappreciated service, and $10 went to a middleman who suffered, at best, a callus on his writing finger and a temporarily sweaty ear from prolonged close contact with a telephone receiver.

Eliminating the Middleman

Now we are getting to the purpose of this book, which is eliminating the middleman. Forget the $8 the patient saved. It's gone. A growing number of practitioners from the solo small-timer to the large group megaprovider are looking towards reclaiming that $10 going to third party administrators. At least, they would like to share in some of those dollars, and add that revenue to other monies gained through new efficiencies and new services with the net result of taking home $7 or $8.

For decades, the insurance companies held a tight reign over the administrative dollars lost by the dentist. Their immense power made it impossible for the dentist to ever even consider trying to regain control. But now, in light of changing attitudes, the door is open. Alternative financing systems of various kinds cracked the wall and created new opportunities for the providers to get into the act.

Maybe you'll lose 20% or so. Don't think of it that way. Change your attitude. Think about the 80% you will gain that you didn't have before.

Reevaluating Profits

Let's discuss how some of those "lost" revenues can be reclaimed. One method may be too obvious to mention. You must cut costs!

Most dentists think they have their fingers squarely on the pulse of their practices, but if they were honest, they would probably admit that even with their expert management, some things have gotten sloppy. A few dollars fall through the cracks now and then. You meant to correct those little problems, but just before vacation it was hard to get your mind clear enough just to handle the patients. So, you planned to take care of a particular problem as soon as you got back. When you returned, it took a couple of days to sort of reprogram your mind for the day-to-day dental delirium. And the next thing you knew—well, you get the point.

If we're going to think about prepaid plans as an 80% increase, with some cleaning up of our routine practice management, staff utilization, and supply acquisition, we might be able to add a percent or two to the figure and gain even more.

There are varying degrees to this cleanup process. On the simple end, you can make sure that whoever orders your supplies shops around a little. Sure it's nice when that representative from the dental supply house visits your office every week. He more or less monitors your inventory for you and makes it very easy to order things. It is nice to have him around to get parts or to provide service when you need it. Take a look at the true cost of that luxury. Are there some things you could buy somewhere else? If you look, you will be amazed at how much you can save by being prudent. There is really no need to abruptly sever your relations with your supplier. Do it gradually.

Simple cleanup, that's the conservative end of cost controls. On the other end you can change the way you run your office altogether. One very successful capitation practitioner in the Sunbelt runs his chain of offices in a very efficient and unique manner. He has no hygienist! He has thousands of patients, several locations, at least a dozen associates, and not one hygienist.

In this dentist's offices patients are not booked with the dentist. They are booked with the dental assistant. The dental assistants have schedules —not the dentists. When a patient comes in the office, the assistant immediately takes any necessary x-rays, and gets them into the developer. This dentist argues that he and most other dentists can clean teeth faster and better than any hygienist. He uses a lightweight air-driven ultrasonic scaler. He checks each tooth as he cleans it, and discusses routine treatments with the patient, chairside, saving that valuable time usually lost while everyone stands around waiting for the dentist to come and "check" the recall patients. If a simple class II is needed for example, he will anesthetize the patient and finish cleaning their teeth while it takes effect. It is conceivable that a patient could get a filling, x-rays, cleaning, fluoride, and a consultation in less than an hour. Patients love not having to come back again. They also love having the dentist clean their teeth. For some reason they perceive his services to be superior. They get an opportunity to talk to him at least. Meanwhile in another room, an assistant is taking temporary impressions for a crown, and so on.

It is not the purpose of this book to tell you how to control costs. The examples given are only to demonstrate the extremes of cost controls. They might not work for you. The point is that increased efficiencies are mandatory for a successful program. Cut costs any way that seems appropriate for you.

Paid in Advance

Let's examine some of the other reasons for changing attitudes. First of all, take a look at the word *prepaid*. It tells you something all by itself. Any business guru will tell you that being paid in advance is the best way to be paid. Countless articles have been written on the subject of collecting money from patients. Conference rooms in hotels across the nation have been totally refurbished a dozen times by the revenue earned from day- or even week-long lectures given to dentists to help them get the money from the patients. Accountants have languished over, and finally cubbyholed, all those accounts receivable in the appropriate little columns, to satisfy the IRS. And still, dentists lose money constantly to patients who pay slowly or not at all.

Paid in advance. It's the best way to keep that 10 or 15% of uncollected dollars off your books each month. If you are smart, you will insist that the patients pay their copayments on the day of the services, thus saving the cost of carrying them each month like you may be doing now. Add the dollars up, and combine it with the money earned by efficiency, and your overall return looks better already.

Selling the Dental Commodity

Dentistry is a commodity just like any other commodity. If you want to stay in business, you have got to sell it. It wasn't like that in the days of too few dentists and too many toothaches, but it has been like that as far back as the memory of just about any working dentist can go. Sure, there are things like professional ethics and clinical appropriateness, but the bottom line is the same as it is in any other business—sales! Take a look at the way success is measured in a dental practice. The key word is *production*. Indeed, many have gotten rich today by selling seminars on how to increase your practice to the $600,000 dollar level or some similar figure. No one gives seminars on doing only what is necessary until you starve to death.

The almost overwhelming overhead of the modern dental practice places increased pressures on dentists to sell. If they don't, they will not generate enough income to even have the chance to be ethical or clinically prudent. They'll be driving trucks. The emphasis, whether dentists will admit it or not, is on finding something to do on each patient that comes through the hygiene department. Practice management consultants are forever talking about marketing, raising your production levels, adding associates or expanded duty interns, hygienists, new and more equipment —sell, sell, sell!

It's tough! And sometimes selling gets in the way of itself. Patients do not like to have something wrong with their teeth each and every time they go to the dentist. They want to think their teeth are well-cared for. They are not dumb. They have heard that dental disease is decreasing overall. Why do they always need this or that done? Many have found another dentist because the one they had been going to found too many things wrong. They figured he was just trying to pay the rent, and they may have been right. This can be particularly difficult for the younger practitioner who takes over the patients of someone older.

If you are not a natural salesman, which many dentists are not, sales can be an additional hardship in an already difficult profession. Again, courses and articles abound designed to make patients accept your treatment plans—"closing the sale" as people in the business world call it. Even if you are the best dentist in the world, if you don't have an office with patients sold on the fact that they need your work, you will never get an opportunity to be that good.

If you have received your money in advance, or at least part of it, some of that pressure to sell, sell, sell, is released. Capitation plans are probably best able to provide this type of mental security. The dentist gets his capitation fee each month whether the patient elects to have any treatment or not. Indeed, he gets the money even if the patient never comes in at all! It sounds like the perfect job everyone is looking for. You get paid for not working. Unfortunately, it is not quite that simple as we will see later. This very concept has been one of the primary issues that has given capitation a bad name. Opponents of capitation have said that the dentists involved have no incentive to provide quality treatments to patients because they would have to actually do something, and that raises costs, and that means loss of money.

It Takes Time

Well, there is no point in denying it. There have been some abuses in the capitation industry. There have been some capitation companies and capitation dentists who have flat gone out of business. The question is: was that a result of a consumer-mandated action as well? You simply cannot treat patients or consumers improperly and get away with it for very long. That is a caveat that applies to any business. Practices like postponing treatments for as long as possible just to take the money today, will catch up with you in the long run. Wise, successful capitation providers know that the real goal is to end up with a patient base floating around in the recall system not really needing any treatment because all of their problems have been addressed. They pay their premiums and require very little other treatment. Here is where the true advances in preventive dentistry can be most advantageously applied, both for the benefit of the patient and the dentist.

The problem is that it takes time. Another fundamental of business is that you must make a deposit before you make a withdrawal. You have got to invest some time in the beginning of the program to get the participants' teeth in a state where they will be stable during the recall phase. That may cost some money at first, but later you will be able to reap the benefits of that patience. If you do not treat the patients right in the first place, they will not feel much like sticking with the plan, and, that means no sign-up in the second and third years where the program begins to get profitable.

The point, though, is worth driving home. The prepaid concept takes the overall emphasis off continual selling. It can be like someone suddenly lifting a 50-pound sandbag off your shoulders.

Other Advantages

We've talked a bit about changing your attitudes towards the financial aspects of establishing prepaid plans. If that's all there were to it, it might not be that attractive. But it isn't! Fortunately, there are other advantages to establishing a prepaid dental program.

The first and probably the most important—even more important than the increased revenue—is the influx of new patients. Can you remember when dentists had these things called "closed practices"? They actually got so cocky that they refused to see any new patients, and were certain they could make it for eternity on the ones they already had. Think about it. Patients still come in and ask if you are accepting new patients. You have to try to conceal your excitement, don't you?

It's a brand new ball game today. In light of the incredible competition coupled with all of the other factors squashing the life out of the profession, you need all the new patients you can get! Indeed, consider the preponderance of data thrust at the practitioner in an effort to address just that single issue—attracting new patients. From newsletters to seminars, everybody is trying to teach you how to get them, and how to hold on to the ones you already have. Remember in dental school how they taught you to tell a patient who comes in fifteen minutes late to go home? You can't very well do that now, can you?

If you can set up a prepaid plan of your own, you will attract a whole flock of new patients. Show them how capable your office is at handling their dental needs, and they will send their friends to you! It's that simple, and that kind of advertising is light years ahead of any newsletter, or internal marketing plan you can buy. Who knows? They might even send someone your way that has a 90% dual-indemnifying plan.

The dental profession is changing faster than Calvin Klein fashions. Most of the changes are for the good, but a few bad ones are eating away the foundation of the profession. One is the attitude of dentists to one another. To use a cliche, it is a dog-eat-dog world out there! You can try to change that, but until the tides of supply and demand correct the situation again, it may be impossible. Or, you can fight them. Every tooth you fill under a prepaid plan is one your competitors didn't. Whether you like it or not, the concept of prepaid dental care is here. If you don't start some prepaid plans, one of your competitors will. And then you'll see what foot the shoe is on.

Give it a Try

Most of the people you sign up under your dental plan, at least initially, are going to be those people who have not previously had any type of dental coverage. They are that 50% you always hear about who do not seek dental care. Are there really any mothers out there who want their kids to have dental problems? It's doubtful. Many don't go because they simply cannot afford it! It rips the heart out of most dentists to see a kid suffering with the rampage of dental caries in a world where that particular problem is now on the run. Many dentists have been known occasionally to do some reparative work on a child without the slightest hope of ever getting paid for it. Call it nobility or whatever. If you have an affordable plan these people can join, you can at least recoup some of your losses.

Keep something else in mind about prepaid plans. It is not an all-or-nothing proposition. Many practitioners have been reluctant to get involved in prepaid dentistry, because they are afraid of becoming a "capitation dentist." Just because you treat some capitation patients doesn't mean you have to give up your fee-for-service practice. Indeed, you're betting that some of those capitation patients are going to send you even more fee-for-service patients. The two are not mutually exclusive.

The big wheels in the prepaid industry will tell you that the name of the game is volume. That's probably true. Take in huge amounts in premiums and hope that a percentage of the participants don't use the program, and those who do won't need or get that much, and you have profit. It doesn't have to be that way. Start small. Take a few small groups and get your feet wet. Make your mistakes and then move on to bigger and better ventures. Then, if the chance for big money in the capitation game comes your way (you've got just as good a chance as anyone), you'll be ready.

It is critical that you change to fit the times. Failure to do so will result in total loss of control over your profession, your practice, and your life. Most experts agree that these types of plans will dominate the 1990s. Blue Cross and the Delta corporations know it. They have gambled millions by setting up their own prepaid plans in an all-important attempt to remain competitive in a changing market. You have to do the same, and you won't if you don't try.

Consider this. In the year that Babe Ruth set the baseball home run record, he also set the strikeout record. If he had been a dentist, certainly, he would have taken a swing at the slow curve the world of money is sending the dental industry. So give it a try. Who knows, maybe you'll help put the power back where it should be—in the hands of the provider.

Chapter 2 What's Available?

Cutting out the middle man and attracting new patients stand out as the most appealing reasons to consider starting a dental plan of your own. Perhaps you know of an employer/employee group which has no existing dental plan. Perhaps you already treat some of those patients. You would probably see them and their friends more often if you could somehow provide them with a means of affording your services. Don't you get tired of hearing what poor businessmen dentists are? We're talking about creating your own market here. That's pretty heady business stuff! Nine basic methods (with a few variations) exist for getting the dollars out of the wallets of the patients and into the hands of the dentists.

The nine basic methods are:

1. Fee-for-Service
2. Indemnifying Insurance
3. Dental Service Corporations
4. HMOs
5. IPAs
6. Capitation/Closed Panel
7. PPOs
8. Self-Insurance
9. Direct Reimbursement

Fee-For-Service

The first is the best. Fee-for-service. What a great concept. You provide a service or a product to someone and they pay you for it on the spot. Wait a minute. Isn't that the way the rest of the world works? Well, not so in dental care. Pure fee-for-service has been on the endangered species list for quite some time. And, although it has been mutated, diluted, divested, and molested, it can still be seen here and there between the trees of the health care forest. Some patients exist who realize the value of quality personalized dental care. They consider it a priority and pay for it. But, the numbers are too small. When you have 90% of the dentists trying to attract 10% of the population, something has to give. Look at your own practice. Certainly, you have some people like this. The problem is that there are not enough of them. And the ones you have don't really need that much treatment anymore if you have been doing your job right. Right?

But fear not. Later in this book, you will understand how fee-for-service could stage a comeback, ensuring its place in the future.

Indemnifying Insurance Carriers

The second method of providing ways in which the groups of patients you have identified can pay for your services is to start an indemnifying insurance company. Let's look at the word *indemnifying.* The dictionary says it means to compensate (a person, etc.) for loss or damage sustained, or to make good a loss, or to give security against future loss or punishment. Insurance companies take in premiums and agree to take the risk of paying for a patient's dental work if the need arises.

They succeed at this because of what is termed actuarial statistics. It's actually an entire science. Statisticians collect massive amounts of numbers as a data base. They keep track of things like the total number of patients between the ages of X and Y, who live in area Z, with incomes of so many dollars, with education levels of such-and-such, and so on. It is extremely complicated. The actuarial scientists provide the insurance companies with a risk factor for each individual procedure they indemnify. Through another series of complicated formulas the insurance companies determine rates that will, according to the statistics, render them a profit over the course of time. In essence, you might say that when you pay your insurance premiums, you're betting that you are going to need that root canal someday, and the insurance company is betting you won't. They have it figured out pretty well and win the bet most of the time. But don't worry, we've got them in the end, because the life insurance companies (most of whom provide dental indemnity) are betting that we won't die, and we are betting that we will. We know who will win that one, don't we?

Since most dentists can boast at least a vague familiarity with the basic insurance concept, let's briefly summarize:

Indemnifying Insurance Summary

Definition

Traditional insurance companies agree to reimburse patients in the event they require some sort of treatment in the future. They agree to take this risk in return for premiums paid, based on mathematical statistics, which predict the frequency with which a certain event occurs. These are called actuarial statistics.

Delivery Setting

Patients under this type of system have total freedom of choice over which practitioner they will visit. Therefore, this method is used in every office environment, from solo private office, to retail group, or in-the-mall facility.

Payment to the Dentist

The insurance companies will usually pay the dentist directly, although they may sometimes simply reimburse the patient for money he pays the dentist. (Most patients don't pay the dentist until after they get it from the insurance company, unfortunately). The insurance companies usually pay a percentage of the dentist's usual, customary, and reasonable fee for a particular procedure, although some plans pay using a table of allowances. Frequently they have plan maximums, and often deductibles that the patient is responsible for up front. Most plans are termed "co-insurance" plans. This means that the insurance company pays its percentage and the patient pays the balance to the dentist. The dentist signs no participation agreement with the insurance company and therefore this contract is strictly between the patient and the insurer.

Advantages For Employer

1. The premium costs of this entire program are known ahead of time. He can choose to pay the entire portion as a benefit to his employees or he can share in the cost and use only a portion of it as a tax deduction. This cost is fixed and can be budgeted accordingly.
2. The headaches of administration of this plan fall solely on the insurance company. The employer only has to send the check.

3. In some cases, insurance companies have set up their own peer review systems and usually have some sort of consulting method to make sure that treatments are appropriate and properly performed, thereby preventing overuse and a subsequent increase in premiums.

Advantages for Patient

1. Freedom of choice of a dentist.
2. Participation in the selection of a treatment plan. Dentists under this type of system may be more likely to provide uncompromised treatments since they assume no financial risk for a particular procedure.
3. Reduced out-of-pocket expenses for patients may mean they opt to be treated more than if they had to pay for the treatment themselves.

Advantages for Dentist

1. Under this system, the dentist does not obligate himself to treat a selected group of patients. He retains the freedom to refer them to other practitioners or refuse to treat them altogether.
2. Financial barriers to treatments are reduced. Additionally, insurance companies for the most part represent good financial risks. The dentist assumes that payment for his services will be swift and definite.
3. Dentist and patient make treatment decisions helping to assure that treatments parallel medical needs.

Disadvantages for Employer

1. If utilization by his employees is higher than anticipated, and the total number of claims paid by the insurance company is above the statistical base, premiums could increase dramatically in the future.
2. Usually premiums have to be paid in a lump sum at the beginning of the contract year. This can be a distinct financial burden.

Disadvantages for Patient

1. Patients still pay co-payments and are responsible for deductibles.

2. Frequently the need for preauthorizations delays treatment.
3. Patients are sometimes lulled into thinking that because they have insurance, all of their dental needs will automatically be covered.

Disadvantages for Dentist

1. In spite of the fact that the contract is between the patient and the insurance company, the dentist assumes the burden of increased paperwork.
2. Dentists complain that sometimes insurance companies imply to patients that any fee above that which is covered by their policies is excessive.
3. Patients assume that insurance contracts are really between the dentist and the insurance company and therefore they are entitled to services without any risk for payments and disputes.
4. Since they have insurance, patients believe that anything they need will be paid entirely by the insurance plan and are sometimes discouraged when they find out they have to absorb some of the financial burden.
5. Fees and plan limits are determined by the insurance companies. Dentists have no input into these decisions and are sometimes unhappy with them.
6. Not all treatments that have been agreed upon by the patient and the dentist are approved of as proper for the patient by the insurance company. Dentists dislike having a third party who has not examined a patient clinically make treatment decisions from x-rays read in distant offices.

In fact, it is even more complicated than we have made it seem. Many more factors need to be taken into consideration in addition to actuarial statistics, including international money rates, and sophisticated investments in world banking. The indemnifying insurance industry literally rules the world, and you can't break into it.

Dental Service Corporations

A third way in which dentists get money for their services is through contracts written and administered by dental service corporations. Ostensibly, they pilot their ships in pretty much the same way as the indemnifiers. They calculate their rates using actuarial statistics. They have premiums, co-payments, determinations of benefit methodology, and various means of controlling the number of dollars they expend on claims each year. There are, however, a few differences in the way they furl their sails.

The first difference is that the dental service corporations were initially organized with the dentist in mind. They were organizations funded by the dentists, and since dental societies set them up, they were administered by dentists. That concept has changed dramatically over the years. The fact that dentists fund these organizations is still true. They do so through research and development dollars. It used to be upwards of 5% of each claim paid. It is now something like 1%. But over the years, those percentages have accumulated and now the dental service corporations have huge sums of money in pools—money which came from dentists. What has changed? Now, fewer dentists are involved in making decisions for these corporations. Economic conditions have mandated that they be run by "business people" rather than dentists, and over the years, fewer and fewer dentists sit on the boards of the dental service corporations. It is ironic that in the participation agreements, dentists agree to continue to provide treatment to patients covered under the contract, even if the service corporation goes out of business! They agree to provide services even if no promise of financial reimbursement exists.

Dental service corporations like the Delta plans and the Blue Cross/Blue Shield plans have fallen into disfavor with many dentists around the country. Many have opted to discontinue their participation in the Delta plans altogether. This is not news. Some of the policies of the dental service corporations have aggravated some practitioners, and most have some sort of story to tell illustrating their dissatisfaction.

These giants of the health care industry, by mandate, are supposed to be non-profit. They have enjoyed a tax-exempt status for years (although changes in the new tax laws may change that). This not-for-profit calling card suggests that they should charge lower rates since they do not have to show a corporate margin of profit like the indemnifiers, who readily admit that they are in business to make money. Somehow the rates do not adequately reflect the discount a consumer would hope to see. What happened to the extra money? As you might guess, dental service corporations are reluctant to discuss that. They say that their rates are as high as those of regular insurance companies because of all of the internal policing they do (participant agreements, auditing procedures, and the like). They claim this ensures higher quality service and justifies their rates. Some Deltas have set up funds to help educate dentists in some of the new technologies being developed in the dental industry. It's ironic that while they are willing to educate dentists in new procedures, they often have no patient contracts which will pay for their services. But they have the fund, and it draws investment interest.

This type of provider discontentment, coupled with the incredible pressure of a changing market, has forced some of the dental service corporations to reevaluate their traditional methods of doing business. Many of them have read the handwriting on the wall and have developed their own prepaid programs in an effort to remain competitive.

None of this really matters anyway, because setting up one of these almost unnaturally complicated monsters is about as difficult as starting your own insurance company, and probably isn't worth the trouble.

Let's look at a quick summary of the dental service corporation concept.

Dental Service Corporations Summary

Definition

Dental service corporations are, for the most part, very similar to indemnifying insurance companies. They determine their rates using actuarial statistics just as the insurance companies do. The major difference in their legal status is that they are non-profit. These companies usually have contractual arrangements with dentists who agree to treat covered patients for pre-filed, usual, customary, and reasonable fees.

Delivery Setting

As with the regular insurance companies, patients covered under this type of plan have total freedom of choice when choosing a dentist. Therefore every office setting is appropriate. They may even choose a dentist who does not participate in the contractual arrangements of the dental service corporation. If so, they may end up paying higher out-of-pocket expenses, but often will receive something from the carrier as well.

Payment to the Dentist

1. *Participating dentist.* The corporation pays the dentist directly just as in a traditional insurance setting. Payment is based on the dentist's customary and reasonable fees, but is limited to a ceiling determined by the corporation. A participating dentist must sign an agreement formally obligating himself to the terms of the corporation contract.
2. *Non-participating dentist.* In this case, patients pay the dentist directly for his services, and the corporation then reimburses them. Since payments are paid to the patient at the median level of reimbursement instead of the 90th percentile, if the dentist's fees are significantly higher than those of a participating dentist, the patient may receive less than he would if he went to a participating dentist.

Advantages for Employer

1. Same as with traditional insurance companies.
2. Higher degree of control of dentist fees through participation agreements and internal audits, thereby reducing risk of dramatically increased fees.
3. Theoretically, costs of peer review and internal controls are borne by the dentist's R & D dollars and therefore rates should be lower. (Controversy exists as to whether or not this is true.)
4. Suggestion of reduced rates since the dental service corporation is non-profit. (Again, this is controversial.)

Advantages for Patient

1. Same as with traditional insurance programs.
2. Dentists agree not to charge the difference between their fees and the corporation fees to the patients.
3. Patient has greater assurance that the fees he is being charged will be closer to what the industry is charging as a whole because of participation agreements.

4. Internal peer review systems theoretically ensure a higher standard of care.

Advantages for Dentist

1. The dentist retains the ability to select, dismiss, or refer patients.
2. He can expect reliable processing and payment of claims just as with traditional insurance companies.
3. The program encourages utilization of dental care.

Disadvantages for Employer

1. The dental service corporation assumes financial risk (which may be passed on to employer) because of higher numbers of claims.
2. The dentist may provide more services than are actually necessary.
3. Rates may reflect the need for internal controls such as peer review and auditing.
4. The non-profit status may deceive the dentist into thinking that fees are discounted, when in reality they are not much different.

Disadvantages for Patient

1. Patient may still have to pay deductible or co-pay for services.
2. Patient is responsible for the total amount of the bill to a non-participating dentist although some of those costs may be refunded by the corporation at a later date.
3. Dentist is tempted to provide more services than are actually necessary in an attempt to increase profits.
4. Patient may feel pressured into choosing a participating dentist rather than one of their own choice because of perception that monies paid by corporation may be lower to a non-participating dentist.
5. Some treatments may be restricted by limitations established by the corporation with regard to frequency and necessity.

Disadvantages for Dentist

1. A percentage of the payment the dentist would receive is retained by the corporation as a provision of the participation agreement as R & D. These funds are used for corporate capitalization purposes such as the purchase of re-insurance from other insurers, and new buildings for the corporations. Some claim that funding for internal auditing and peer review come from premium dollars, others claim it comes from R & D.
2. The field auditing done by the corporation may disturb the normal functioning of the office causing lost revenues. Additionally it is viewed as an invasion of privacy by some of the practitioners.
3. The same patient problems arise as with traditional insurance programs. Patients think the contract is between the insurance company and the dentist and therefore they are not involved in any of the disputes. They think that if they have insurance, all of their claims are paid in full and are unhappy to find that they may have to pay for some of the services themselves.

HMOs and Their Cousins

For now, let's give up on the first three money-delivering systems: fee-for-service, indemnifying insurance, and dental service corporations. It is very unlikely that developing one of these systems is feasible for an individual entity. Let's take a look instead at what you could do.

Let's talk first about capitation plans, and more specifically, about their first generation children, HMOs. But wait—shouldn't it be the other way around? Isn't capitation the method HMOs use to convey funds from the consumers to the practitioners, and therefore aren't the HMOs sort of the parents and capitation plans the children? You might say that, but if you look at historical fact, you can trace the capitation concept back much farther than the formal HMOs. Indeed, one investigator, in a paper from the Health Maintenance Organization office of the Department of Health Education and Welfare, claims to be able to trace the idea back to the 19th century. In 1931, employees of the city of Los Angeles and their families could pay dues of $2.00 per month and receive a wide range of medical services, including hospital services, at the Ross-Loos medical group. The Ross-Loos experiment is still in operation today, and is now licensed under the HMO

Act. The underlying payment methodology of this plan is capitation, and since the plan has survived for so long under this system, it has no doubt suffered more intense scrutiny than any other program.

The concept of collecting fees on a per patient basis in advance of performing any treatment (capitation) can be difficult to investigate. Early capitation plans were born in the trade and labor unions. Interpersonal relations within these groups were sometimes private matters, held together by bonds of trust which remained unbreakable. Briefly, a practitioner would approach the leader of the union and ask if he could provide services to the members for a monthly fee and a discounted fee schedule. The leader of the group would grant permission and even help to promote the plan among the members. He, of course, expected to retain a certain fee, thereby subjecting himself to criticism for conflict of interest, if anyone found out. Consequently, in-depth investigation of the early days sometimes leads to closed mouths and dead ends.

In the beginning prepaid programs were, for the most part, initiated in unions and remained in that realm for years. It isn't like that anymore. Obviously, capitation programs have spread very rapidly. And while the fact that Douglas A. Frazer, past president of the United Auto Workers, sits on the board of directors of Metropolitan Independent Dental Associates (a Detroit-based prepaid dental company) demonstrates how involved unions remain with prepaid plans, capitation is now available for people in all walks of life.

With the capitation format well established, it didn't take very long before the concept had proliferated through just about every facet of the health care industry. Unions set up their own clinics providing everything from out-patient surgery to eye wear. Today of course, most of the major hospitals in the country are involved in some sort of PPO or HMO program.

It is the mandate of the government to govern. Practically everyone has at one time or another been forced to shelter his personal business from the prodding long arm of the law. With the advent of capitation, the tectonic plates of change were tearing at the foundation of traditional health care delivery systems with incredible force. Legislators couldn't resist! In 1973, in response to the diligent efforts of Paul M. Elwood, a physician from Minnesota, they passed the first HMO law. They amended it in 1976, 1978, and again in 1981. Its provisions for capital acquisitions made it possible for an explosive expansion of prepaid health care in this country.

HMOs are changing the face of health care in a way not felt since the discovery of bacteria. The HMO Act of 1973 and its subsequent amendments rule the HMO industry, and provide the basis for rules and regulations of all health care plans today. After passage of the federal acts, most of the state legislatures passed similar laws. Today, most of the dental capitation plans (as well as other alternative dental delivery formats) are governed directly, or in some cases loosely, by these HMO laws. Rules relating to company organization and contractual arrangements with subscribers in general were spawned by the HMO Act.

Let's take a look at this all-important regulation to try to get a feel for the kinds of things that will be important later. The law, for those of you who wish to examine it in more detail, is cited as:

Health Maintenance Organization Act of 1973
U.S. Code 1982 Title 42 280c, 300e et seq.
Dec. 29, 1973, P.L. 93-222, 87 Stat. 914

Health Maintenance Organization Amendments of 1976
U.S. Code 1982 Title 42 300e et seq.
300n-1, 1395mm, 1396b
Oct. 8, 1976, P.L. 94-460, 90 Stat. 1945

Health Maintenance Organization Amendments of 1978
U.S. Code 1982 Title 42 300e et seq.
1320a-1, 1396a, 1396b
Nov. 1, 1978, P.L. 95-559, 92 Stat. 2131

Health Maintenance Organization Amendments of 1981
U.S. Code 1982 title 42 300e to 300c-4,
300e-4a, 300e-6 to 300e-9, 300e-11, 300e-17, 300m-6
Aug. 13, 1981, P.L. 97-35, 95 Stat. 357 940 to 949

The HMO Act

Using the citations above you can easily obtain copies of these regulations from any law library. The Health Maintenance Act says the following:

A Health Maintenance Organization (HMO) is a legal entity which:

1. Provides its members with basic health services for a basic health services payment.
   a. The payment shall be paid on a periodic basis without regard to the dates the services themselves are rendered.
   b. The payment shall be fixed without regard to frequency, extent, or kind of health service (within the basic health services) actually furnished.

c. The payment shall be determined by a community rating system, except in the case where the services are provided to a full-time student attending an accredited institution.

d. The payment may be supplemented by additional nominal payments for the provision of specific services unless those payments are determined to be a barrier to the delivery of those services. These additional payments shall be fixed.

2. An HMO may provide supplemental health services to its members for a payment in addition to the payment for basic health services. This supplemental payment will follow the same guidelines defined above for the basic payment.

3. An HMO does not have to provide services under its contracts to patients for an illness or an injury that would be covered under workmen's compensation.

4. If services are provided to one of its members who is covered additionally by an insurance company, the HMO may charge the insurance company for payment.

Within the context of the HMO law, basic health services are described as:

1. Physician services (including consultant and referral services by a physician)

2. Inpatient and outpatient hospital services

3. Medically necessary emergency health services

4. Short-term (not to exceed twenty days) outpatient evaluation and crisis intervention mental health services

5. Medical treatment and referral services (including referral services to appropriate ancillary services) for the abuse of or addiction to alcohol and drugs

6. Diagnostic laboratory and diagnostic and therapeutic radiological services

7. Home health services

8. Preventive health services, including imunizations, well-child care from birth, periodic health evaluations for adults, voluntary family planning services, infertility services, children's eye and ear exami-

nations conducted to determine the need for vision and hearing correction

9. Any other services the Secretary of Health and Welfare determines applicable at a later date and formally publishes in the Federal Register

The service of a physician is expressly defined as service rendered by a physician, a dentist, optometrist, podiatrist, or other health care professional.

Supplemental services are defined as those services that could be rendered by a dentist, optometrist, podiatrist, optometrist, or other health care professional.

The Health Maintenance Act provides specific organizational requirements as well as specific ways in which treatments will be delivered. The act specifically states that: (1) Unless the treatment is very unusual or infrequently used, or, (2) Unless the treatment is provided under strict emergency conditions where conventional HMO methods can not be used because of the immediate need for the treatment, the services of an HMO will be delivered through:

1. Members of the staff of the HMO
2. A medical group or groups
3. An Individual Practice Association
4. Physicians or other health professionals who have contracted with the HMO
5. Any combination of the above

This outline of how the services of HMOs will be delivered has led to the terms *Staff model HMO*, *Group model HMO*, and *Direct-contact model HMO*.

Dentists function in all of these combinations today, either by working directly within the HMO on a part- or full-time basis, or by contracting to provide services out of their own offices through an IPA or through direct-contact contracting.

Further, the act states:

1. Providers in the HMO shall, within the area for which the HMO has contracted, provide basic health services with reasonable promptness, and in a manner which assures continuity.
2. Services contracted for by the HMO, when medically necessary, will be available twenty-four hours a day, seven days a week.

a. If an HMO has a service area which is primarily non-metropolitan, it may make services available outside its service area, if that service is not a primary care or emergency service, or if there is an insufficient number of providers in that area to deliver such a service.

b. The HMO will reimburse expenses to a member who has to receive treatment outside the treatment area if that treatment is medically necessary and immediately required.

And of course, the legislators felt obligated to throw in a joke. They said that if your entire facility is wiped out by a natural disaster like an earthquake, or a nuclear war, all you have to do is make a reasonable good-faith attempt to deliver the services. That's nice.

The Assumption of Risk

The major concern of the federal and state legislators (and later of the individual state insurance commissioners) is the assumption of risk. What the governing agencies are afraid of is that an entity like an HMO or a capitation company will take dollars from the members and then not be able to provide the services, or go out of business altogether, and abscond with the funds. Take note of this assumption-of-risk principle—it is very important because it is the basis of many disputes in the prepaid industry, and the foundation of legislation. Here are some of the things the HMO Act says about the assumption of risk:

1. Each HMO shall have a fiscally sound operation and adequate provision against the risk of insolvency.
2. Each HMO shall have satisfactory administrative and managerial arrangements.
3. Each HMO shall assume full financial risk on a prospective basis for the provision of basic health services.
4. The HMO may obtain insurance or make other arrangements for the cost of providing to any member basic health services, the aggregate value of which exceeds $5,000 in any year.
5. The HMO may obtain insurance or make other arrangements for the cost of basic health services provided to its members other than through the organization because medical necessity required their provision before they could be seen by the HMO.

6. Obtain insurance or make other arrangements for not more than 90% of the amount by which its costs for any of its fiscal years exceed 115% of its income for such fiscal year.
7. The HMO may make arrangements with physicians or institutions to help absorb some of the financial risk on a prospective or anticipated basis for the delivery of basic health services.

Numbers 6 and 7 refer to the concept of reinsurance. We will discuss it more later. In addition to these rules established by the legislature to insure that the HMOs assume their risk appropriately, they have also laid down some other organizational rules. They said:

1. The HMO may enroll persons who broadly represent the population in terms of age, social group, and income.
2. If the HMO is in a medically underserved area, the HMO may carry only 75% of its enrollment from the medically underserved population, unless that population is also in a designated rural area.
3. The HMO may enroll members who are also entitled to Medical Assistance under a state plan approved under the Social Security Act
   using methods approved by the Secretary of Health and Welfare.
4. The HMO may not expel or refuse to re-enroll any member because of his health status.
5. If the HMO is a private organization,
   a. One-third of the members of its governing body must be made up of members of its organization at large.
   b. Its governing body must have equitable representation of members of the underserved population served by the organization.
6. If the HMO is a public organization,
   a. It must have an advisory board to the governing body of the organization of which one-third of its members are members at large of the organization.
   b. This advisory board must have definite policy-making authority for the organization.
7. The HMO must have a method for resolving grievances between itself and its members.

8. The HMO must have a method for assuring quality control over the treatments it provides, and it must have means of following through on the treatments offered to assure that they are successful, in other words, a peer review system.
9. The HMO must have methods to insure its members that they will not have to pay fees that are legal obligations of the HMO.
10. The HMO must have contractual arrangements with hospitals that are regularly used by the HMO ensuring that its members will not be liable for any fees that are by law the obligation of the HMO.
11. The HMO must have adequate insolvency insurance.
12. The HMO must have adequate financial reserves.
13. The HMO must also demonstrate acceptable means of collecting and reporting statistics regarding its operation and utilization to its members and to the public in general and must make such reports available annually.

The HMO Act of 1973 is an enormous monster. Its unedited version is a couple of hundred pages long. This is the quintessence of its being, although to understand it fully, a much more thorough study must be undertaken. It is of utmost importance because it is from this essence that a whole new genre of health care phenomena will germinate, dominating the horizon of medicine well into the next century. The individual points of inception and operation outlined here will serve as a model for many of the remaining topics in this book.

One interesting sidelight should be mentioned. The federal government will give you a grant (if you apply and are accepted) of up to $75,000 to do a feasibility study to see if an HMO is warranted in a certain area. In addition, if it is deemed that an HMO could be effective in a given area, the federal government will give you up to $2,000,000 to start your HMO in the form of actual grants (you do not have to pay them back) or in guaranteed loans. It is conceivable that you could apply for such a grant for dental capitation as well, providing that you could supply adequate justification for your program. Obviously, legislators consider the HMO concept a viable one for the future.

Closed Panels

Somewhere during the genesis of prepaid systems, the term *closed panel* was born. It serves as an underlying criterion for defining any prepaid system. Closed panels are groups of providers to whom patients under any alternative prepaid plan must go to receive health care services. HMOs deliver their services through closed panels. Capitation programs are manned by closed panels. Even the providers in a PPO are, when strictly interpreted, closed panels. This is one of the most significant differences between these types of systems and traditional treatment modalities. It is also the spear point of contention that opponents of the prepaid plans throw at the public. Freedom of choice is their defense to an ever-increasing assault upon their pre-set livelihood.

The IPA

The HMO Act of 1973 outlined another entity under which dentists can receive money for their services. It is the IPA or Independent Practice Association. The HMO Act says:

> The term "Individual Practice Association" means a partnership, corporation, association, or other legal entity which has entered into a services arrangement or other legal arrangements with persons who are licensed to practice medicine, osteopathy, dentistry, podiatry, optometry, or other health profession in a state and a majority of whom are licensed to practice medicine or osteopathy . . . .

The American Dental Association defines IPAs as:

> Legal entities organized and operated on behalf of individual participating dentists for the primary purpose of collectively entering into contracts to provide prepaid dental services to enrolled populations. Dentists may practice in their own offices and may provide care to patients not covered by the contract as well as IPA patients.

An IPA is a group of dentists who get together and form a separate entity (usually a corporation) that contracts with the HMO to provide dental services. The IPA has an agreement with the HMO, and a separate agreement with the contracting dentists to provide services directly out of their individual offices. This is the primary method HMOs use to staff the *group model.* The IPA receives payments from the HMO, and then it pays the dentists according to the terms of the provider contract. Usually, the IPA receives a lump sum per capita each month. They then pay the dentist on a monthly per capita basis as well. If the utilization of the plan is higher than expected, the IPA may show a loss, and its individual providers will suffer by sharing in that difference. On the other hand, if utilization is low, then the IPA will show excess, and theoretically this will be distributed back to the dentists.

Some IPAs may agree to pay their providers a percentage of their usual customary and reasonable fee. For example, let's say the IPA pays 80% of the dentist's fee to him. They will hold 20% in reserve to protect the IPA from overall high utilization. If at the end of a given contract period, there are funds remaining in the reserve pool, they are distributed to the dentist on a pro-rata basis.

A dentist providing his services on an IPA basis is not limited to treating only patients from the HMO system. He may treat patients from other IPAs or from capitation companies, or private patients as well. The last time anybody checked, back in 1981, the typical practice providing services to an IPA treated only 5 to 20% IPA patients. The remainder were traditional patients of one kind or another.

Capitation

The discussion of the HMO and IPA concepts leads directly to a discussion of capitation companies. HMOs contract with groups of individuals, or with employer/employee groups to provide services in return for advance payments. They then pay the dentists for the services using one of a variety of systems. The capitation company does exactly the same thing. The difference is that the capitation company is usually owned and operated by private individuals who determine policy independently, with little input from dentists.

The capitation company establishes contractual relations with the individual dentists, and then goes directly to employers to solicit their business. Once their system of providers is in place, the capitation company may contract with an HMO to provide services in the same manner as the IPA. Theoretically they could contract with an IPA to provide services using their network of providers to fill-in gaps in the IPA system, so that contractual arrangements are fulfilled. The point is that the capitation company can contract with any purchaser of its services. In each scenario, some of the dollars that should flow from the patient to the practitioner are kept by the capitation company management for their services.

The concept is simple, but as you might have guessed, it has grown complicated in practical application. As far as anyone can remember, the first capitation plan was started in California by a dentist named Max Schoen. He and his friend, Dick Naismith, entered into an arrangement with the children of the West Coast Longshoremen's Union, in 1954, about the same time as the first Delta program was being started in the same area. Dr. Schoen in his office in Los Angeles, and Dr. Naismith in his office in San Francisco, operated a pure capitation program. They didn't even have an intermediary company. The plan was administered directly out of their offices. A similar program, based on the principles Schoen delineated, opened in the same time period for the Hotel and Restaurant Workers of Los Angeles.

Later, separate legal entities began to administer capitation plans, and their popularity increased. They were operated in what was called the "pure" form. The subscribers, members, or purchasers—whatever you would like to call the patients—paid their money monthly to the capitation company. The capitation company took their percentage out and paid the dentist an amount based on the numbers of patients who had signed up for his office, again on a monthly per capita basis. Soon however, capitation companies began to notice increased numbers of complaints from some dentists and not from others.

The problem? Some of the providers—those who had patients signed up for their offices but never saw them—were receiving the capitation fees each month, but not treating any patients. These practitioners had reached economic Nirvana. They had accomplished the goals of workers since the beginning of time. They were doing absolutely nothing and getting paid for it! On the other hand, some practitioners were experiencing a very high utilization of their services, and in effect, were carrying the entire risk burden for the services of the whole provider group. For some reason they didn't like that. Many dropped out of the program as soon as they could to begin licking their capitation wounds. That gave the entire capitation industry additional bad press and made it difficult for managers of the programs to solicit the services of dentists to take their place.

Risk Pools

A solution came in the form of a bastardized blend of pure capitation and fee-for-service dentistry, called the modified capitation plan, or the risk pool program.

A few of the premises are the same: The patients pay the capitation companies either directly through payroll deductions, or through employer contributions as part of a benefit package, or through union dues, or whatever. The capitation company takes its administrative fees off the top, as usual. The remainder is distributed to the dentists. Predictably, it is the distribution to the dentists that is altered. Each member is paid a monthly per capita rate based on the numbers of patients who sign up for the program, as in the pure system, but a portion of the total amount of money collected from the patient is saved by the capitation company and placed into a pool. Individual dental procedures are given a unit weight which is determined by a variety of methods. At the end of a given payment period, each procedure performed by an individual dentist is converted into units. The units are then divided into the pool dollars and the dentist is paid for the numbers of units performed. And—because nothing can be simple—minimums, maximums, and separate pools of money for orthodontic work are added to make things complicated.

The risk pool is intended to blunt the economic blow from one office to another and to reduce the incentive for abuse of the program. A dentist who is losing money may find it difficult to make decisions based strictly on medical necessity, keeping economic factors from entering into the equation.

There you have it. Capitation. It isn't that new. It isn't that original. It isn't that scary. And surprisingly, many feel it may already be a doomed species with other new and different plans evolving from the primordial ooze of health care. Let's look at a quick summary of closed-panel systems.

Closed Panels Summary

Definition

A closed panel practice is established if patients eligible for dental services are required to visit a limited number of dentists at a limited number of locations.

Delivery Settings

1. *Single Clinic.* All services are provided at one central location, usually an office administered by the capitation company or some other administrative group directly affiliated with the employer group.

2. *Multiple Clinic.* Same as above, but usually with more than one location. HMOs are frequently established in this manner.
3. *Independent Practice Association.* Individual dentists or groups of dentists contract with providing agency to provide services in their individual offices.
4. *Private Office.* Contracted for by direct contact HMO model and capitation company.

Payment to the Dentist

1. Monthly payment based on a per family amount less administrative fees.
2. *Fixed-fee schedule.* A table of allowances is set up for an individual piecework type service.
3. *Modified fee-for-service.* Dentist receives a percentage of his fee. If funding of payment pool is insufficient, dentist may receive less than he normally would.
4. *Pre-payment in full.* Dentist agrees to accept a certain amount to treat a certain number of patients no matter what they need. There may be contractual arrangements where individual patients pay additional fees for services they alone may require.

Advantages for Employer

1. Perception of lower premiums when compared to fee-for-service programs.
2. Worries about over utilization and the subsequent increased premiums are reduced because the dentist bears the risk of providing services.
3. By considering an alternative system, employer sets up a competitive bidding situation between various entities.
4. Patients receive a dramatic decrease in out-of-pocket expenses, and the perception of the program is one of better benefits given by the employer.

Advantages for Patient

1. Many co-payments are eliminated, reducing out-of-pocket expenses.
2. All services are responsibility of dentist, including referrals for specialty services.
3. This type of system usually offers expanded hours and more staff.
4. No paperwork is required, and there are no additional costs.

Advantages for Dentist

1. Predictable monthly income assists in budgeting of finances.
2. There is an influx of new patients and the subsequent hope that they will refer new patients who may not be enrolled in the program.
3. Dentist can control the type and frequency of services provided.
4. Little processing of claims is necessary.

Disadvantages for Employer

1. Peer review may be unavailable and when it is available, it is handled by the administrator.
2. Until recently, plan administrators may have been outside the jurisdiction of insurance commissioners.
3. Premium dollars may actually be buying a reduced level of care, because the dentist may try to cut costs by not offering service, using inferior products, and laboratory services.
4. The use of consultants by traditional delivery companies to determine the appropriateness of care is eliminated.

Disadvantages for Patient

1. Treatment may be spread over a long period of time to allow premiums to catch up with treatments rendered.
2. An overall lower level of care may be provided as more expensive treatments are eliminated.
3. Peer review may be eliminated.

4. Patient may have to pay for some treatments in the form of co-pays.
5. Patient loses freedom of choice of dentist.

Disadvantages for Dentist

1. The dentist accepts the financial risk of treating the patients who sign up for his office, thereby becoming the insurer in the system.
2. Referral to specialists may have to be paid for by the dentist.
3. Dentist loses the ability to accept or reject cases since he has agreed to treat all of the needs of the group of patients who enter his office.
4. Dollars from the patients are filtered first through plan administrator.
5. High volume of patients tends to favor larger group practitioners over the small solo office.

PPOs

The immutable laws of evolution which govern all changes in nature apply equally in business. A need arises. An opportunistic species develops to satisfy that need. Time—the almighty mitigator of all things—asserts its undeniable influence, and soon the gradient of change forces permutations and adaptive radiations. Those businesses with few complaints on the part of its clients or staff remain and proliferate. Those who cannot change to meet the requirements of the economy and the whims of the public, die out.

The HMOs and capitation plans are tiny fledgling creatures in the time span of health care, yet they have met with considerable controversy and adversity. Some observers think it may already be time for massive changes in their business methods. Certainly, it is time for them to move over and share the waters with a new species. The PPOs swim confidently and grow strong on the stolen eggs of the pure HMO plans.

PPO stands for *Preferred Provider Organization.* The American Dental Association likes the terminology *Contracting Dental Organization.* They say "preferred provider" may lend undue support for one provider over another on the basis of skill as opposed to purely financial considerations described by their various contracts. Basically, a PPO is established when a practitioner or group of practitioners enters into an agreement with some sort of group of potential patients to provide services to that group at reduced rates. In return for the reduced rates, the group of patients publishes the name of the provider to its members and those members are thereby encouraged to visit the office of those providers within the PPO. You might say it is a closed-panel system in that regard, and technically you would be right. The two systems are different enough, however, to warrant separate classifications.

PPOs are popping out of the ooze faster than frogs after the first warm spring rain. Two of the earliest dental PPOs were The Insurance Dentists of America (IDOA) and The Connecticut General PPO. The Connecticut General PPO has met with some unfortunate environmental circumstances. It had contracted with a Denver-based management firm, United Dental Network, whose job it was to provide dental offices for the system. The appropriate axiom here is: "Pigs get fat. Hogs get slaughtered." United Dental Network charged dentists an initial franchise fee of $500, a monthly administration fee of $500, and marketing fees of $400 to $800 per month. In addition, the dentist had to agree to accept fees from patients of this system that were 15% lower than his usual, customary, and reasonable fees. We know cost containment has to come from the dentist, but this was extreme.

The system did not produce the tremendous influx of new patients into the offices that it was supposed to. Certainly it was not enough influx to justify these types of charges. The dentists, even with their universally alleged lack of business acumen, pulled out of the system. Connecticut General pulled their contract with United Dental Network, and UDN went bankrupt. It was a shaky start for dental PPOs. A spokesman for Connecticut General at the time said they intended to continue their push into the alternate delivery market, and that they still felt it was a viable proposition for the future.

IDOA, on the other hand, did far better with a less stringent set of guidelines for their participating dentists, and is still in the market today enjoying participation with a host of insurers. Under this system, PPO providers are allowed to join with no fee. The PPO then contracts with the insurance carriers. The carriers offer their reduced fee schedule to the providers, who either accept it or reject it. If a provider rejects too many fee schedules, he will be dropped from the system. The fees are usually 15–20% lower than prevailing usual, customary, and reasonable rates. The insurance companies usually look to sign 20–25% of the providers in a particular area, and then publish their names to the patients contracting with the system as providers who will grant the reduced fees.

Since the patients have to visit the offices of the practitioners involved with the program to receive the reduced fees, it is a closed-panel system.

The major difference goes back to the old "assumption of risk" principle. The patient is not paying anything up front to the dentist for him to assume the responsibility of treating all his dental needs. The only risk is that if the dentist is not efficient enough to make a profit with the reduced fees, he will go out of business. If that happens, the patient has the option of going to another dentist in the system, without having to pay any additional fees. Because there is no assumption of risk, the PPO concept is currently driving the government regulators nuts. They can't find anything to regulate. Consequently, the rules and regulations governing the activities of PPOs are, in most places, non-existent, or loose, at best. We will see how we can use this to our advantage later.

While PPOs look like they may rule health care much in the way the dinosaurs exerted their dominance over the planet for 130 million years, their path is not totally free of obstacles. The PPO has met with some antitrust problems. Arguments have been shouted from both sides of the fence. Some say the discounted fees of a PPO constitute price-fixing and therefore violate the principles of the Sherman Antitrust Act and/or the Clayton Act. Some have said that health care did not come under the jurisdiction of the acts in the first place. The Supreme Court, in *Arizona* v. *Maricopa County Medical Society* ruled that health care was indeed to be governed by these acts and treated like any other industry. Yet in 1983, the Federal Trade Commission issued an advisory opinion stating that the "co-operating provider program" of Health Care Management Associates based in New Jersey did not constitute a price-fixing arrangement, nor would it violate the FTC act. The antitrust waters are very choppy right now, but it looks as though they will calm enough for the PPO concept to sail majestically in the future. One basic concept when developing a PPO in light of the antitrust controversy is not to sign up every practitioner in the area. Keep it limited. Then your PPO will be in the position of collectively competing with all of the other providers in the area, and the antitrust question will be more difficult to prove.

Another obvious problem from the provider standpoint is that the PPO takes another slice out of the health care dollar pie before it gets passed to the dentist. The insurance company takes a piece, the PPO takes a piece, and the dentist has to discount his piece as well. But here may be where the solo practitioner or the small group has the advantage in the long run. If the individual provider goes to the employer and offers a discounted program, theoretically he should be able to provide greater discounts and thereby eliminate two of the middlemen! You don't charge them "premiums" as do the insurance companies, but rather, "membership fees," similar to those charged by any other purchasing club, like the ones the credit card companies offer. To receive benefits at the discounted rate, members must come to your office or the office of one of your associates. That's it exactly! One club of dentists makes an arrangement with another club made up of patients. It is probably the most viable option for the individual practitioner or small group to offer pre-payment plans to purchasers independently. It is even better than capitation!

PPO Summary

Definition

A preferred provider is an individual practitioner or a group of practitioners who join together and offer discounted services to a group. The group advertises the names of the providers to its members.

Delivery Setting

Private or group offices.

Payment to the Dentist

1. This is basically a fee-for-service program. The dentist agrees to accept the fees of the PPO or the underwriting insurance company as payment in full.
2. The patient still pays co-pays and deductibles to the dentist.

Advantages for Employer

1. Theoretical reductions in premium costs.
2. Administration of program by third party.
3. Utilization review procedures may be performed.

Advantages for Patient

1. Patient may have freedom of choice if enough dentists join the program.

2. Patient may move freely from PPO to non-PPO dentist and pay the difference in co-pays.
3. If patients go to the PPO dentist, they may have lower out-of-pocket expense.

Advantages for Dentist

1. PPO should advertise dentist's name to members of the group.
2. The ability to dismiss and select patients still remains.
3. Decisions relating to type of treatment remain with the patient and the dentist.

Disadvantages for Employer

1. If an insurance company is involved, the insurance company is assuming the risk. If higher than anticipated utilization of the program exists, employer will be charged higher premiums.

Disadvantages for Patient

1. Patient has to pay deductibles and co-pays.
2. Patient may have concerns about standard of care since dentist is receiving less money than he ordinarily would.

Disadvantages for Dentist

1. Dentist receives less money for services provided.
2. Patient assumes that insurance contract is between doctor and the insurance company and therefore any disputes will be settled between them.
3. Plan administrators control fee limits.

Self-Insurance

A self-insurance plan is exactly what the name implies. The employer assumes the role of the insurance company and assumes the financial risk of the program itself. This type of program is funded by the company directly through its treasury or through some sort of trust fund. The company may pay claims based on a table of allowances with its employees paying the difference between the table fee and the usual, customary, and reasonable fee of the dentist, or it may pay a fixed percentage of any dentist's fee. The employer may perform all of the administrative functions or hire an outside management company to administer the program. This type of arrangement is known as an ASO or *Administrative Services Only* contract.

This can be a risky proposition for the employer company. If utilization is high, they could get burned very easily. In which case, they will have the option of (a) absorbing the losses and their consequences, (b) reducing the coverages, or (c) dropping the program altogether. Employers can buy "stop loss" insurance from various companies to insure them against financial insolvency in the event the program's expenses exceed treasury or trust fund limits. This is similar to the reinsurance that HMOs and indemnifying insurers use to back their programs and protect them against miscalculations in their utilization expectations.

These programs have been popular lately, especially for smaller companies who have been deemed not cost effective in terms of administration expense by the large third-party carriers. Let's summarize.

Self-Insurance Summary

Definition

An employer indemnifies its employees for dental services by setting up a fund and paying the dentist directly or through an ASO contract with another insurance company.

Delivery Setting

Total freedom for the patient in choosing a dentist means this method can be used in every office type.

Payment to the Dentist

The dentist is paid on a fee-for-service basis. He gets his money in part from the company through claim checks and part through the patient in co-pays and deductibles.

Advantages for Employer

1. If program is administered directly by the company, administration fees may be lower than with any other type of arrangement.
2. No advance lump sum premium payments to other companies.
3. With ASO contract employer retains control over pre-authorizations, usual, customary and reasonable rates, treatment review, and fee verifications.
4. Program can be used by any type or size of employer.

Advantages for Patient

1. Freedom of choice of dentist.
2. Participation in selection of treatment.
3. Higher level of treatment because dentist has no financial incentive to hold back services.

Advantages for Dentist

1. Dentist retains ability to dismiss or accept patients.
2. There may be a decreased need for pre-authorization.
3. Treatment decisions are made by the dentist and the patient.

Disadvantages for Employer

1. Depending on how much paperwork and record-keeping company does, administrative costs may not be less than with traditional means.
2. Company is assuming the risk for the finances of the program.
3. If employer administers program, it may be difficult to control cost and quality.

Disadvantages for Patient

1. Patient may still be responsible for considerable out-of-pocket expenses.
2. Patient may have no cost controls or quality assurance programs.

Disdvantages for Dentist

1. If the program is administered as ASO agreement, dentist may have increased paperwork.

Direct Reimbursement

This is the program that has been officially supported by the American Dental Association. And why not? It is the closest thing to fee-for-service imaginable. The patient pays the dentist and then is reimbursed by showing a receipt to the employer. It is the consumer who has dictated this entire epoch of change within the health care industry. The employer is paying the bills, but where are the advantages to the employer under either the self-insurance or the direct reimbursement systems? The employer assumes all of the risk and is entitled to no fee reductions in any way at the payment end. True, he can negotiate with employees for limits and reimbursement parameters, but that puts the burden of health care back on them, and that is the one place they do not want it. Since it is clear that the consumers make the decisions in the long run about how business will be run, this program seems to be in line for some serious environmental hazards. It may have to modify and adapt rapidly or jump on the endangered species list before it ever really gets going.

There is no need to summarize this program. It is exactly the same as the self-insurance concept, except that no insurance company or administrative company is involved. The disadvantage to both the patient and the dentist is that since all of the treatment expenses are out-of-pocket to the patient, treatment services may not be available because the patient may not be able to afford them—just like in the old days.

Closed-Panel Direct Reimbursement

We have defined nine methods of getting money to pay for dental services. In light of the discussions of self-insurance and direct reimbursement, we should talk about a tenth, possibly a hybrid. While it does not have an official position regarding it , the ADA has already coined a term for this hybrid. They call it "closed panel direct reimbursement."

Let's say a certain company has established a dollar amount they are willing to give to their direct reimbursement plan in a certain year. Now, a sharp businessman goes to the employer and says, "If you instruct your employees to go to my office exclusively, I will agree to charge you 20% less than the going rate for a service or treat your employees according to a fixed table of allowances that you and I will agree to, or I will agree to pay back a certain percentage into your fund at the end of the year after I have collected interest on it for a few months."

And so we have it. The early stages of evolution unfolding before our eyes. Others are beginning to see the handwriting on the wall. Companies have already gone out and more or less hired a dentist to service their employees for a fixed yearly amount. One city in Illinois, in which one large corporation was the major employer, reportedly advertised for a dentist to come to provide services to the entire community for a fixed yearly salary. Now that's about as closed a panel as you can get. The company pays the dentist and the patients can choose to go to him for essentially nothing or go to the dentist of their choice and pay whatever his fees are. The idea works because so many unions and groups of employees have been forced to give up many of their benefits (just to hold on to their jobs) that they are willing to settle for this type of arrangement instead of nothing at all. It looks as though this trend is here to stay for awhile, especially if large employers have anything to say about it.

Obviously, it is almost impossible, and certainly impractical, for you to set up your own insurance company or dental service corporation. However, it is just as unlikely that in the future you will be paid strictly on a fee-for-service basis either. That leaves the HMO/capitation/IPA model, the PPO model, and the direct reimbursement/self-insurance models. You could help an employer to establish his own direct reimbursement or self-insurance plan, but unless you are certain that you will end up seeing most of his employees either by convenience or by contract design, what good will it do? You may be able to convince your colleagues to set up an IPA and then find an HMO willing to participate with you, but it isn't easy. We will look at that again later. What's left is the self-directed capitation plan or the PPO and its derivatives. The balance of this book will be devoted to investigating these two alternatives.

A quick tip to you small solo practitioners interested in providing a few small contracts to some of the groups in your immediate area: skip the capitation part and jump directly to the PPO model plans. The states have recently made it very difficult (although not impossible) for the solo practitioner to offer capitation plans like you could only a short time ago. They no longer want you to assume the risk you have been assuming indirectly for years. The fast track for you is to present a discount program to that small company. You'll get your piece of the prepaid pie and you'll need a smaller dose of antacids later.

Chapter 3 Separate the Entity

If you want, you can start a dental plan and operate it directly out of your office just like they did when they started the first plans. You might come up with a catchy name like "Dr. Dan's Dental Plans," or something similar. You could sell it to every group or individual that happened to knock on your door. But don't! Set up a separate company and try to keep your name out of it.

Establishing Credibility

One of the major hurdles you are going to have to overcome when you begin this type of business is a distinct lack of credibility. Unless you want to remain a real mom-and-pop operation with groups that contain only two or three members at a time, you will find it very difficult to compete with the multitude of alternative delivery carriers. Enticing groups with 25 to 50 members will be extremely difficult. You can forget groups with 50 to 100 members altogether. This is a legitimate business that has the potential of generating a respectable income for you. "Dr. Dan's Dental Plans" just doesn't get it! The problem of credibility will haunt you like the plague when you are first beginning this type of venture. Insurance commissioners will wonder about you, as will employers, potential patients, and other practitioners. It is important to do everything that you can to offset this handicap.

The Limits of Your Professional Corporation

As your experience with prepaid dental plans grows, you will begin to see a variety of reasons (in addition to the need for credibility) for setting up a separate administration company. Let's look at few. If your dental office is organized as a professional corporation (P.C.), technically it can not enter into any other endeavor besides delivering the services of your particular profession. Check with your lawyer, but if push came to shove, it could be argued that you are in violation. If you own a separate corporation, that corporation could own real estate, enter into contracts with groups, enter into contracts with other providers, buy businesses, sell businesses, sell toothpaste, advertise, purchase tax-deductible equipment like computers and other office supplies, share utility costs (in your home, for example), pay your rent, hire staff, provide tax deductions for office space, pay for educational trips, pay for autos for salesmen who have to drive around soliciting business, enter into contracts with suppliers for discounted merchandise, enter into contracts with laboratories to provide lab services, set fee schedules different from the ones in your office, pay you management fees as though you were an independent contractor, entertain prospective clients, and generally participate in a whole slew of activities difficult to justify in a P.C.!

Now, stop for a minute and reread that last paragraph. Spend a little time thinking about it. Soon you will see other reasons to start a separate corporation.

Geographic Realities and Adding Providers

Selling prepaid plans can be a lot like owning a boat. At first a 16-foot runabout is fine. Soon you graduate to an 18 footer. Next comes the 24 footer with the cabin. You outgrow that soon and find yourself looking at those 35-foot monsters with flying bridges and sundecks. It won't be long before you uncover a potential group that has more members than you can handle. More specifically, they won't be able to handle you. You may have sufficient office space and chair time to accommodate the extra load, but the problem often will not come from that direction. If your office is the only provider in the system, groups may not wish to sign up with your program, simply because it is not convenient for them to travel to your location if it is too far. A firm rule for this cannot be found. In rural areas, distances between offices can be as much as 25 miles. In the city, distances of only a couple of miles may be too far. One provider in Arizona is able to sell to groups with members that live as far as 50 miles from his offices. As you explore guidelines established by the HMO Act and other acts passed by the individual states, you will find that decisions regarding licensing are influenced by geographic location and service area as well as other criteria. It becomes a question of relativity, but the point is that you may find yourself in the position of turning down a group because of inability to service them geographically. You will be faced with finding another location, or finding another provider to help you to service them.

If that is the case, it will be very helpful if you are set up as a separate corporation. If you own multiple offices of your own, all spaced sufficiently to handle the needs of the people in your groups, so much the better. But, if your plan is successful, sooner or later you will find it necessary to solicit the services of providers other than yourself in order to compete. They will not want to jump on your bandwagon, if it looks as though they are working for you and your office and not for their own.

Remaining Anonymous

You will find it convenient to remain anonymous and the corporate front is excellent for that. Many patients want to think of their doctor as someone exclusively dedicated to health care. They do not want him to be involved in business, and they would like to think that he spends any time away from the office reading and studying dentistry. Many dentists have helped to nurture this image, and have avoided admitting that they are in business to make money, just like everyone else. Therefore, it may not seem appealing to some dentists to have to go out and sell dental plans. The perception may not uphold the image. On the other hand, no one would object to you sitting on the board of directors of a separate corporation involved in some sort of insurance business. Appearances are important. Directing the activities of an outside corporation selling dental insurance plans sits better in the minds of patients than Dr. Dan hawking patients out of his office.

Remaining anonymous has other advantages. Prepaid plans by their nature create a certain perception in the minds of patients and doctors as well. It is the perception of a discount. For some reason, in spite of the fact that a discount is what everyone is looking for, this perception conjures up negative reactions. Patients may not want to associate with a dentist who gives discounts. If you are offering discount dental plans directly out of your office you may occasionally encounter this type of reaction. On the other hand, patients do not mind if you participate in some plan offered by an outside company. Indeed, you may have already had people ask you to participate in a plan so that they could take advantage of it and still visit your office. It happens all the time, and why this difference exists is anybody's guess.

No matter which type of plan you end up offering, there will be rules that must be followed in order to assure your success. Some of these rules may not be popular. If you are the guy making the rules, your popularity may be affected. It is easier to hide behind the cloak provided by a separate corporation, and say, "I'm sorry Mrs. Jones, but your dental plan only covers such and such." This way it is the other guy making the rules and not you. Patients seem to accept this much better, and let's face it, you do that very thing today with the conventional payers you deal with. The inevitable shortcomings of any plan involving doctor and patient can be mitigated by a third party. Admittedly, it is a small point, but on a day-to-day chairside basis it can relieve a lot of stress.

You could call these points ethical considerations. There are no clear-cut rules about this,and chances are likely that no one will ever start some sort of litigation over the whole matter, but generally speaking,you will find it much more relaxing to separate yourself from the plan as much as possible.

Money Flow

There are some clear-cut rules about taxes, finances, and the way you are paid, however. One of the reasons you are considering starting a prepaid plan yourself is to regain some of the health care dollars stolen from providers by third party carriers and administrators. What difference does it make whether you are paid totally in relation to the services you provide, or partly by the services you provide, and partly by the premiums or membership fees given to a company you own? The answer is taxes and

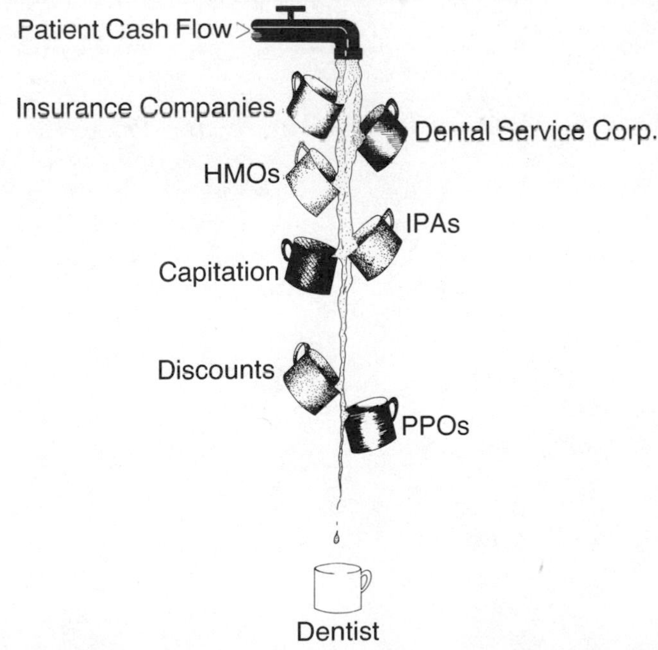

salaries. You're nodding your head, and if you're thinking you should consult your accountant and tax attorney about this, you're right.

Let's take a look at the flow of dollars from the patients to the doctors.

It can be viewed as a triangle with whoever is paying (employers or patients) at the top, the insurance companies (or other third parties) at the lower left corner, and the dentist (or provider) at the opposite corner. The dollars flow out of the patient's pockets to the insurance company in the form of premiums, and to a lesser extent to the dentists in the form of co-pays. The money then flows to the dentist from the insurance company. In most practices, this is the predominant source of cash. The co-pays which the patient pays directly to the dentist are usually lower than the money that is paid by the insurer. This is due simply to the nature of the contract, or to the fact that patients frequently fail to have those procedures provided which are not reimbursed by the carrier at a high level. The bad part is that the dentist has no control over the money that flows to him from the insurance company, and it is the main source of his income. If the dentist assumes the role of the third party carrier and takes over that position in the triangle by virtue of his involvement in a company that contracts directly with the patient, he can effectively regain some control over the dollars coming from that leg of the flow. By control over co-pays in the contract, he also exerts some control over the flow of cash that comes directly from the patient as well. So, with control over cash coming from different directions, it is time for some "creative accounting."

When the money flows directly into the dental office either from an existing insurer, or from the new company the dentist puts in place, it must be treated as ordinary income by his dental office. This means it must flow through all of the internal programs of the office, like profit- and pension-sharing plans, for example. Depending upon the tax status of your practice, this may or may not be advisable. The point is that now you have control where before you had none. You can decide where the money should go. Maybe you would like to have some of the money paid directly to you as a salary from the new prepaid company, with the appropriate withholding and other taxes removed. Perhaps you would like to have it paid to you as a "consulting fee" or "management fee." You can then treat the income as personal rather than corporate, and make the best tax decisions. Obviously, you will want to ask for help from your accountant. But to repeat, you have created more options for yourself. If you ran the program directly from your office, the income you received would be ordinary income to the practice. No options. No flexibility. No creativity!

The Float

Let's take a look at an interesting sideline about cash flow. It's called "floating." No, not the kind of "floating" a veterinarian does to the molars of a horse when they get so sharp he can't eat. It's the kind of floating banks do with billions of dollars, to make millions of dollars—invisibly. When you drive up to your local bank's drive-in window and make a deposit, the bank does not instantly credit your account with the cash. They wait a day or two to see if the check you gave them is good. The vast majority of the checks they receive are good and not very risky for the bank. Because of that, the banks don't just let the money sit in some drawer somewhere—they invest it! Yes, even for two days. Let's say they take in a million dollars in deposits on that day, and invest it for only 8% somewhere. If you do the arithmetic, you'll see they make about $438 in two days using someone else's money, with little risk. Actually the amounts invested are far greater, and so are the times and the percentages, but you get the point. Money makes more money if managed correctly. If your dental office does not need the cash immediately, you can run it through an interest-bearing account owned by the prepaid company, and you can do whatever you like with the interest. And since we are speaking about creativity, let's let our imaginations go crazy for a minute. The best advice is to start these plans slow and keep them small, but say just by accident you sold a contract to an employer who had one thousand employees, and was willing to pay your prepaid company $25 per head per month for their dental premium, so you would take in about $300,000 a year. Let's say too, that he paid those premiums on the first day of each month, and you contracted with other providers to do the work (obviously too much for a solo practice). If you agreed to pay them on the thirtieth of each month, you would have about twenty-nine days to use the money. If you made a conservative investment of 8% as in the example above (and you probably already know how to do better), you could receive as much as . . .. Well, you get the idea. It doesn't work too well with very small numbers, or in situations where there are creditors involved who are charging more interest than you could make investing conservatively, but this is how the big boys do it, and there is nothing wrong with putting the necessary mechanisms in place so that you can do it later if you should happen to get big in a hurry.

Growing Pains

That brings up one more argument in favor of setting up another company to administer your prepaid program. What if Dr. Dan should get lucky one day? What if he finds a large group who would like him to provide services under a prepaid contract? Should he decline based on the advice given here about staying small? Of course not! If that's your situation, go for it! But if you do, you might suddenly find yourself with a business that is more valuable than the dental practice ever could be. What if someone wants to buy you out? It sure would be nice to be able to sell it without encumbering the dental office as well. That kind of speculation on the future goes farther still. Suppose, in order to win a contract, you have to be able to provide services in a location where, even with your network of providers, it would be impractical for you to operate, or you are asked to provide services that you are not capable of offering. You might have to make arrangements with another company to provide those services for you—a merger of sorts. Who knows what kinds of arrangements will evolve in the future. You may want to weave your network of providers into another network to accomplish a common goal. You may have to offer more than one type of contract to the same group in order to compete. All of these speculative scenarios are better handled by a separate company rather than just Dr. Dan's office.

Government Intervention

Still not convinced? Then consider one more thing. Not too long ago, you could offer just about any plan you wanted out of any office setting. The governmental regulators, insurance commissioners, and the like, did not care. Some did not have clear power to regulate these types of plans. Many had the enabling legislation, but were not enforcing the rules. Whatever the case, you could operate the plan if you wished. Not so today. More and more states have passed laws restricting the activities of prepaid companies, and most states are now enforcing them. Soon they all will be, and one thing that looks doomed is the ability to operate one directly out of an office. It may not be illegal, but it will be impractical. Why not read the handwriting on the wall? Don't try to set sail in this complicated sea of alternative payment with the tiny tub of your office as a vessel. Get yourself a yacht! Set up a separate company which will be more capable of weathering the inevitable storms to follow.

Company Format and Business Basics

You should be convinced now that forming a separate corporation is the best course to follow if you are serious about setting up a prepaid dental plan. The first thing you will need is a new name that doesn't necessarily reflect the involvement of your practice with the management of the company. Remember the credibility problem. Try to choose a name that will reflect a degree of sophistication. Instead of Dr. Dan's Dental Plans try something like Dental Management International. For our hypothetical discussion we will use the name "DMI plans."

The next (and probably most important) thing you should do is to have another meeting with your lawyer and your tax accountant. You will have to decide what type of company you are going to form. Should it be a d/b/a? Should it be a limited corporation, a full corporation, a public corporation, or what? It really doesn't matter much if you intend to keep it small and just offer services out of your office or perhaps with a limited number of associate providers. If you foresee the possibility of expanding sometime in the future, you may want to adopt a corporate format which will permit you to divide up some shares and give some of them to others. As we shall see, this may become important later if you want to offer a formalized provider participant PPO-type plan.

There is some sound advice in the suggestion that you form your company under this corporate umbrella for malpractice reasons as well. If prepaid providers are linked in any other manner other than via the corporation, there can be some argument that each is liable for the actions of those other providers with whom he associates—liability that may arise from actions involved with the delivery of the actual services. In other words, if one of your unincorporated comrades commits malpractice, you could be held liable as well. Since we are talking about liability, forming a corporation makes sense from an economic standpoint as well. In the event of insolvency, stockholders of a corporation can only be held financially liable for the amount of money they have directly contributed in the form of stock acquisitions. Reducing one's overall financial liability makes sound business sense.

For now let's assume it is a regular sub-chapter C corporation, and avoid Chapter S status to allow us to decide later what to do with the profits.

Your accountant can help you in this regard and can provide the necessary papers for formal corporation. The next thing you are going to need is a physical location. Remember, one of the important steps in making this type of thing work is establishing credibility. A mailing address can't hurt. Some state regulations require it anyway. It can be located in your office, your home, or in a separate location. If it is in your home, for example, and is a separate entity, it is okay to allocate some of your heating bills and your mortgage payments to that corporation on a proportional basis. You can even charge it rent if you would like. This is acceptable to the IRS, but they have been known to send a representative out to check if they are nervous about something.

A phone with a separate line would be nice. Remember you want to separate this company from the dental office and from you personally. When it rings answer it "DMI plans," and keep the kids off it.

You'll need some stationery and some envelopes with your corporate logo. Spend a little time on this. Make it look professional. Get a checking account. If you are a corporation, go through the proper licensing procedure in your state and show proof to the bank so that you can deposit your checks without a hassle. If you are going to be a d/b/a, file the appropriate papers at the county seat, and set up the account in your company name. A savings account may be advisable as well.

Computers

Get a computer! This may be a repulsive idea for some. You can run a dental office without necessarily needing a computer, but you can not run a prepaid company without one. We've said that we would like to keep it as simple as possible, and for some of you getting a computer is a step towards complication instead of towards simplification. If you don't already know how to use one, once you become comfortable with the use of a computer, you will see how much one can be used to simplify your prepaid dental effort. They are critical to the management of a small company, and absolutely indispensable to a larger organization.

This is not intended to be a course on computer usage, but it is important to understand what you will be using it for, so that you can buy it prudently. You don't need a huge mainframe. You don't need the most expensive fancy package available. You need an inexpensive one and a compatible printer. A letter quality printer would be best since you will be sending a lot of letters, and they should look as professional as possible. The machine itself is not as important as the software it will use, since the machines themselves seem to be heading towards a certain degree of uniformity anyway.

Having a computer in your office will make many tasks easier. First of all, the computer can be used to file or index the patients who choose to participate in your plan. They will have to be filed according to the usual name, rank, and serial-number type of information. They will also have to be cross-referenced according to the group they belong to and to the effective date of their coverage. Any simple filing system can handle this for you, right off the shelf so to speak. You will find that it will not be hard to use either.

You will also need a method for tracking patient payments. If you are dealing with one large employer/employee group which pays once a month for all of its members, this will obviously not be too difficult. If however, you contract with an association or other group situation in which the individual patients may pay their own premiums, you will have to know who paid and who didn't. The computer will tell you instantly. In most cases, the same filing system you use to index the patients and groups can be used to track these simple financial arrangements. You will have to send statements monthly to these people, and you will find that the filing program can do that as well.

Next, you will want to produce promotional material, descriptive and informational material, plan proposals, update letters, solicitation letters, provider contracts, group contracts, and a host of other written material, including the paperwork necessary to obtain a license. So, you will need a simple word processing program. It would be nice if your filing system and your letter writing system were compatible so that you could personalize your correspondence, but it isn't necessary. There are many ways of getting around this. But it is simple to link the two systems, so why not do it? Your filing system will be able to print mailing labels for you, which will make billing and most of the other communication problems simple. If the filing system can't handle it, the word processing system will. The labels are an invaluable labor-saving device.

Still down on the computer? When you think about it, you can handle the entire business with two canned programs; a filing system and a word processing system. What could be simpler?

Set to Go

So, we've filed the proper papers to be in business, either corporate, or DBA. We have all this stationery laying around with "DMI Plans" stamped all over it. The phone is hooked up. We have a computer humming away over here in the corner. We've got some checks. Why not go out there and sell some contracts? Get some cash to go with the checks. Let's develop a marketing strategy and go to it. But are we forgetting something? Oh yes. Is this legal?

Not really. Not yet at least. Remember, we said that the insurance commissions of most of the states are enforcing the laws with regards to licensing of these programs. We either need a license, or a letter from the insurance office telling us in writing that what we intend to do is okay. In order to get that, we need to know what product we are going to offer. That question, for all practical purposes, boils down to a choice between capitation or preferred provider plans involving some sort of discount.

It may be worth repeating that the fastest way for the smaller solo practitioner to enter into the prepaid market is by concentrating efforts on the discount PPO-modeled plan discussed later in this book. The following section about capitation will be helpful, however, because it is from the earlier capitation concept that most of the rules and regulations for the more modern plans have been derived. A good understanding of the principles of capitation will be invaluable in operating any new venture in the prepaid industry.

Chapter 4 Developing the Product

Developing a prepaid dental business is a function of the blending of five basic concepts:

1. Developing a product
2. Making it legal
3. Developing sound relations with providers
4. Marketing the product
5. Developing sound relations with subscribers

Before you can have even the slightest hope of being successful with this new business, you must be sure that you know exactly what you are offering for sale. "Know your product" has served as a motto for salesmen for years. It is applicable in this endeavor as well.

Capitation as a Model

For all practical purposes, the product will be limited to dental capitation plans, or discount plans modeled after the PPO concept. Of the two, capitation is by far the most complicated. Its licensing and operational requirements deserve special attention, and will serve as a model for establishing rules and operational guidelines for the discount plans to be discussed later.

If we choose capitation as a product, we are basically offering a plan whereby a defined group of individuals pay us in advance for services they may need in the future. They pay us monthly on a per head basis. We distribute the prepaid premiums to the dentists with whom we have contracted to provide services. We receive a limited amount of money in the form of co-payments from the subscribers only when certain services are delivered. If they do not need or use the program, we keep the premiums anyway, and thereby profit. If they elect to use the services, we are obligated to provide them and therefore may lose money, depending upon what it costs us in expenses.

The accepted definition of any organization intending to seek federal qualification as an HMO is:

> . . . any organization, either for profit or nonprofit that accepts responsibility for the provision and delivery of a predetermined set of comprehensive health maintenance and treatment services to a voluntarily enrolled group for a prenegotiated and fixed periodic capitation payment.

Certainly any dental capitation program fits this definition perfectly. Therefore it is easy to see how this type of program qualifies for regulation under the HMO Act of 1973, the subsequent state acts, and the changing enforcement policies of the state insurance commissioners. Before DMI Plans can offer capitation programs to groups of subscribers, you must check with the insurance commission in its state, to see if licensing is required, and then comply with the application procedures for obtaining that license. A list of the state insurance commission offices can be found in Appendix A.

Chapters 5 through 8 will detail further the development of a dental capitation plan and the licensing requirements. To assist you in determining whether dental capitation is right for you, the following summary of how the various states treat prepaid dental plans is provided. It will tell you if a particular state has separate legislation regarding dental plans, if it regulates them under authority of another law, or if it regulates them at all. In addition, wherever possible, it will give the dollar amounts needed to apply for licensure, whether there is a formal application, how much is required for surety deposits, net worth approximations, and other specific qualifications where applicable. In addition, it will give citations of pertinent legislation to aid you in gathering data regarding dental plans in your state.

It is of paramount importance to realize that this summary is only offered in an attempt to quickly familiarize the reader with general ideas about his state's attitudes with regard to prepaid dental plans, at the time of this writing. It should be pointed out that this entire industry is experiencing a great deal of flux, with the various commissions hustling to develop a uniform thinking with regard to this phenomenon. By the time this goes to print, it is conceivable that changes in policy will have taken place. Therefore, one considering the development of such a plan should call or preferably set up an appointment with the insurance commission to outline exactly what they have in mind, and discuss the various regulations that may apply. A good rule to keep in mind is that most insurance offices are willing to consider any plan if it is presented well. You may find that even in a state with stringent regulations you may be able to begin a plan if you present it properly to the officials and are willing to work with them to get it operating. Remember, these are bureaucratic representatives. They are used to complicating things, and thinking in terms of why you cannot do something. You should only focus on how you can! Your task is to convince them. Be persistent.

As you examine this reference, you may find instances where a particular state has outlawed this type of activity, yet you are aware that it exists anyway. The research for this confirms this observation. Some companies are simply operating illegally. Some insurance offices are not aware of all of the activities in their state. Some are, but have been unable or unwilling to start procedures to correct the situation. Companies that are operating illegally risk prosecution. Some are willing to take the chance and may be considering challenging the legality of the regulations in their state. Either way, the financial undertaking might be prohibitive for smaller organizations.

Remember, do not take this summary as absolute!

Summary of State Regulations

Alabama

1. Requires capitation plans to be registered.
2. Has application but does not charge a fee to process.
3. Requires a deposit of a surety bond or marketable securities totalling $50,000.
4. Plan must have minimum working capital of $100,000.
5. Not sure about discount PPO-modeled plan; wants to examine it.

Applicable Statutes: Chapter 21 title 22 Alabama Code.

Alaska

1. Has no separate law governing HMOs or PPOs and nothing specific for dentistry.
2. PPOs must qualify as an insurer, a hospital, or medical service corporation.

3. No clear policy regarding dental prepaid-paid plans.

Applicable Statutes: None.

Arizona

1. Has specific law governing prepaid dental plans.
2. Requires licensing and application.
3. Requires $125 application fee.
4. Requires a $50,000 fidelity bond for all corporate officers.
5. Requires graduated surety bond deposits based on the number of members, ranging from $25,000 to $200,000.
6. Has a financial reserve requirement of 2% of contract amounts.
7. Does not specifically regulate discount PPO-type plans.

Applicable Statutes: A.R.S. 20–1001 A.S. Chapter 23, Article 1. R9–23–110.

Arkansas

1. Does not have separate legislation for dental prepaid-paid plans.
2. Regulates dental plans under general HMO statutes.
3. Requires a certificate of authority after meeting requirements.
4. Requires the combination of premiums, deductibles, and co-pays represent discounts of no more than 25% when compared to conventional insurers' plans, which would practically limit delivery of services to the closed panel.
5. Allows insurers to enter into PPO arrangements.
6. Allows self-funded PPOs.
7. Has no separate PPO laws.

Applicable Statutes: Ark. Stat. Annotated 66–5200, et, seq., Ark. Stat. Annotated 66–3703.

California

1. Regulated by the Department of Corporations.

2. Termed "Specialized Prepaid Health Service Plan."
3. Application with a $2,500 application fee.
4. Requires a fidelity bond of $10,000 to $2,000,000 depending on anticipated enrollment.
5. Requires a surplus tangible equity of a certain amount based on enrollment.
6. After licensing, plan must follow specialized set of rules termed Knox-Keane law.
7. Has no law governing PPOs but wants to examine each case for its individual merits.

Applicable Statutes: Cal. Admin. Code Title 10, Chapter 3, Sub-chapter 5.5, Cal. Health and Safety Code, Section 1340–1399.

Colorado

1. Has separate prepaid law for dentistry.
2. Has application and fee.
3. Requires surety bond.
4. Requires deposit for guarantee of funds.
5. Has reserve requirement.
6. Will consider other plans such as PPO on a per case basis.

Applicable Statutes: Title 10 Insurance Code, Section 16.5.

Connecticut

1. Has separate legislation for dental prepaid plans.
2. Has application with $50 fee.
3. Requires surety bond and/or percentage of premiums deposit.
4. Does not allow single-service HMOs.
5. Will consider discount PPO-modeled plan; has no clear rules.

Applicable Statutes: 38–174–U Connecticut General Statutes.

Delaware

1. Has specific legislation for capitation plans.
2. Application procedure.
3. Requires general surplus fund of 2% of gross premiums for a year to a limit of $50,000.
4. Unique state in that it has developed prepaid dental regulations before it developed HMO regulations. Currently is introducing regulations in legislature for regulation of HMOs.

Applicable Statutes: Chapter 38 of the Delaware Code, Title 18, Chapter 39 Delaware Code.

District of Columbia

1. Has no laws for prepaid dental plans.
2. Does not regulate under any other laws.

Applicable Statutes: None

Florida

1. Has separate law governing dental service plan corporations.
2. Requires specific application and licensing.
3. $225 application fee.
4. Requires $100,000 working capital for every six months of operation.
5. Does not regulate discount PPO-type plans.

Applicable Statutes: Florida Statutes 1983, 637.401–637.429.

Georgia

1. Effectively outlaws dental capitation, or limited panel systems altogether.
2. May allow dentist or group of dentists to offer discounted fee-for-service contracts provided the overall premiums and deductibles do not substantially undercut dentists' normal reimbursement for services, thereby placing him at risk.

3. Insurance office will provide copy of 1982 Attorney general opinion which discusses situation in detail.

Applicable Statutes: Georgia Insurance Code, 56–36 and 56–102.

Hawaii

1. Has no specific legislation for prepaid plans.
2. Is not currently aware of any plans in the state.
3. Has not had experience regulating them.
4. Has law that requires all employers to provide medical insurance for their employees.
5. Regulates HMOs from Department of Labor.

Applicable Statutes: None.

Idaho

1. Has no specific law regarding prepaid dental plans.
2. Interprets some of its HMO laws to apply to dental plans.
3. Wants to encourage development of health care plans that provide readily available, accessible, and quality comprehensive health care to their members as an optional method of delivery, but wants to examine the merits of each plan as it is presented.
4. Has somewhat unusual law that governs the administrators of any insurance-related plan.

Applicable Statutes: Title 41 Chapter 39 Idaho Code, Section 41–3902, 41–3903, 41–3905, Chapter 9 Section 41–901.

Illinois

1. Has no specific law covering prepaid dental plans.
2. Interprets other legislation to cover dental capitation plans.
3. Has strict enforcement of policies, and has recently tested its authority to regulate at the Supreme Court level against a dental capitation plan.
4. Requires $1,000 application fee.

5. Requires working capital of $100,000.
6. Does not regulate plans with no assumption of risk like PPOs.

Applicable Statutes: Ill. Statutes Chapter 32 595–596.

Indiana

1. Considers a dental plan a "Special Service Health Plan," and is currently attempting to amend existing laws to regulate them more specifically.
2. New law calls for an extensive application procedure and scrutiny by the commissioner.
3. Requires a surety deposit of $50,000 or 2.5% of the plan's gross annual fees up to $250,000.
4. Plan must have capital account of $100,000.

Applicable Statutes: Senate bill #192, 27–8–7–1 Indiana Insurance Code, Chapter 7.

Iowa

1. Does not allow dental capitation plans.
2. Allows dental benefits to be attached to a full-service HMO, or offered as a supplemental benefit added to a group health insurance policy.
3. Does not regulate PPOs, but recognizes their existence in the state.

Applicable Statutes: None.

Kansas

1. Currently does not regulate prepaid dental plans, but is considering attempting to have legislation passed in the future.
2. Asks that any company considering offering prepaid service plans subject itself to a review by the insurance commission. All documents, brochures, and other material will be scrutinized. If no problem is found a "No Objection" letter will be issued. This makes it possible to offer discounted fee-for-service plans of the PPO type

without question, but makes it questionable for capitation plans because of their assumption of risk.

3. Companies do not have to comply with the review request. However, they may be subject to fines later if legislation is passed.

Applicable Statutes: Kansas Statutes Annotated 40–3201, et seq.

Kentucky

1. Has specific law governing prepaid dental plans.
2. Has specific application.
3. Requires $600 in filing fees for the application, and an additional $5 for each form filed.
4. Requires a cash deposit of somewhere between $25,000 and $75,000 (determined by the commissioner).
5. Does not regulate PPOs, but requires that the difference between contract provider fees and noncontract provider fees be less than 25%.
6. Does not allow closed panel PPOs.

Applicable Statutes: Kentucky Revised Statutes Chapter 304.43, 806 Kentucky Annotated Review 18:020.

Louisiana

1. Claims to have complete set of regulations for the administration of pre-paid dental plans available for $5.
2. Refers to plans as "dental contractors."
3. Claims that only insurance companies are allowed to offer these plans. No single individual companies or administrators will be allowed to operate one in this state.

Applicable Statutes: Louisiana Statutes, Title 22, Section 1510.

Maine

1. Has no laws governing prepaid dental plans.

2. Has no regulatory guidelines for establishment of prepaid dental plans.
3. Regulates PPOs.

Applicable Statutes: Title 24–A M.R.S.A. Chapter 19, Subchapter II and Title 24–A M.R.S.A. Chapter 32.

Maryland

1. Specifically regulates all forms of dental prepaid plans.
2. Has specific application guidelines.
3. Requires a surplus bond of 7% of the gross contract and certificate income for one year.
4. May require surplus assets at least $75,000 greater than all liabilities.

Applicable Statutes: Subtitle 42 48A 582 Maryland Insurance Code.

Massachusetts

1. Has no specific laws.
2. Is currently in process of developing governing guidelines.
3. Is definitely interested in inspecting plans and has recently contributed to insolvency of one plan operating without authority.
4. Considers prepaid plans as an additional line for existing insurance company, but foresees the possibility of entrepreneurial activity.
5. Not actively seeking compliance from business.

Applicable Statutes: None.

Michigan

1. Does not have separate law governing formation of prepaid dental plans, but interprets a portion of the HMO law to regulate dental capitation.
2. Requires application for licensing.
3. Requires a $1,000 application fee.
4. Requires minimum $10,000 surety deposit.

5. Requires a minimum net worth and minimum working capital assurance.
6. Requires a percentage of contract deposit.
7. Does not regulate discount fee-for-service plan modeled after the PPO concept.

Applicable Statutes: Chapter 333 of the Michigan Public Health Act, Part 210.

Minnesota

1. Has no specific law regarding dental prepaid programs.
2. HMO law does not cover prepaid dental.
3. Has not yet attempted to regulate prepaid dental plans although they are currently considering some proposals.
4. Considers cap plans to be insurance and will request compliance with some form of the HMO law.
5. Does not consider discount PPO-type plans to be insurance.

Applicable Statutes: Minnesota Statutes 62 D.

Mississippi

1. Does not have specific laws for prepaid dental plans.
2. Allows some prepaid plans but only through a chartered insurance company.
3. Has specific freedom of choice legislation which effectively rules out any closed panel system.
4. Unless legislation changes, does not foresee likelihood of single-service company operating in this state, especially if not directed by insurer.

Applicable Statutes: Mississippi Insurance Codes 83–511, 83,41209.

Missouri

1. Does not specifically regulate prepaid dental plans.

2. Has no specific legislation authorizing the operation of dental capitation plans under their HMO law.
3. Dental capitation plans do exist but no attempt to regulate them has been started by the insurance office.
4. PPO-type discount contracts are allowed as well.

Applicable Statutes: RSMo 354.400–354.550 (HMO).

Montana

1. Has no specific legislation for prepaid dental plans.
2. Considers all prepaid plans a form of insurance and regulates them as casualty companies, or under a new plan effective Oct. 1, 1987, which governs HMOs and PPOs.
3. Has an application procedure.
4. Requires casualty certificate of authority with financial reserve of $400,000.
5. If licensable under the new HMO law, financial reserve will only be $200,000.
6. Not sure how discount fee-for-service plan will be treated.

Applicable Statutes: 33–1–201 (5), 33–1–102 (1), Senate bill #371, Senate bill #353.

Nebraska

1. Has specific legislation regarding prepaid dental plans.
2. Requires application and licensure.
3. Requires extensive qualifying examination by the Department of Insurance.
4. Requires a $100 application fee.
5. Requires a $50,000 surety bond.
6. Also regulates PPOs.

Applicable Statutes: Nebraska Revised Statutes Chapter 44–3801 through 3826, Nebraska Revised Statutes Chapter 44–3201 through 3291, Nebraska Revised Statutes Chapter 44–4101 through 4113.

Nevada

1. Has separate law regarding prepaid dental plans.
2. Requires application for licensure.
3. Requires a $530 application fee.
4. Requires a reserve account of 3% of gross premiums.
5. Requires premiums collected to be a minimum of 75% of the expected losses for the plan.
6. Requires surety bonds ($250,000,) fidelity bonds for officers ($1,000,000) and stop-loss insurance.
7. Also requires inspection of PPO plans.

Applicable Statutes: Nevada Revised Statutes 695D, 695C, 686B.125, 679B.152.

New Hampshire

1. Does not have specific regulations for prepaid dental plans.
2. Is not now actively regulating plans.
3. Reserves right to inspect workings of plan to determine if licensing is necessary, but is not seeking organizations to file for application.
4. Has HMO regulation, but does not know of any single-service HMOs such as dental cap plans operating.
5. Has PPO law and is in process of rewriting it in legislature.

Applicable Statutes: Revised Statutes Annotated 420–B, Revised Statutes Annotated 420–C.

New Jersey

1. Has specific legislation regarding prepaid dental plans.
2. Requires application and licensure.
3. Requires 2% surplus over assets of contract premiums to $100,000.
4. Regulates various percentages of contract gross revenue, as to how it will be spent.

5. Limits numbers of practitioners to the number of enrollees.
6. Requires $50,000 fidelity bond on officers.

Applicable Statutes: New Jersey Insurance laws, Chapter 48D 17–48D 1–24.

New Mexico

1. Has specific prepaid regulations.
2. Application procedure with $500 fee.
3. Requires graduated trust deposit depending on number of members. $25,000 minimum for 2000 members or under, increasing to $200,000 for 40,000 members or more.
4. Requires $50,000 fidelity bond on administrators.
5. Does not regulate PPOs.

Applicable Statutes: New Mexico Insurance Code 59A, Article 48, Section 1–19.

New York

Claims "We do not have any HMO or PPO dentistry in the state of New York. Both are considered illegal."

North Carolina

1. Has no separate statutes governing prepaid dental plans.
2. Regulates dental as part of the HMO act.
3. Has application process.
4. Requires a $49 application fee.
5. Does not regulate PPO activity at this time but has recently passed legislation to do so, and is in the process of establishing a set of guidelines for PPO-type plans.

Applicable Statutes: North Carolina Insurance regulations, Section .0300, North Carolina HMO Act Chapter 57B, General Assembly Session 1985 Chapter 735, House Bill 1037.

North Dakota

1. Does not have specific legislation.
2. Is not currently regulating.
3. Has only two plans in existence, one from a dental service corporation, and the other is offered as supplemental benefits by an HMO.
4. Has no clear-cut policy.

Applicaple Statutes: None.

Ohio

1. Has specific prepaid legislation.
2. Has application with a $25 fee.
3. Requires $50,000 surety bond or cash deposit.
4. Requires $250,000 surplus asset fund.
5. Requires $50,000 fidelity bond for administrators.
6. Has PPO legislation pending.

Applicable Statutes: Ohio Revised Codes Chapter 1736, Ohio Administrative Rules Section 3901–1–43.

Oklahoma

1. Has specific prepaid dental legislation.
2. Application with $100 fee.
3. Requires fidelity bond of $50,000.
4. Requires surety deposit based on number of enrollees. For 5,000 members or less, it is $25,000. It reaches a maximum of $200,000 at 40,000 people.
5. Requires a financial reserve of 2% of all gross premium charges up to a maximum of $500,000.

Applicable Statutes: Oklahoma Statutes 1983 Chapter 36, Section 6141.

Oregon

1. Considers all prepaid health organizations "Health Care Service Contractors," and requires licensing.
2. Requires one-third representation on the board of directors by non-doctors.
3. Requires $250,000 surplus or 50% of the amount of average claims.
4. Requires $250,000 surety bond.

Applicable Statutes: ORS Chapter 750.

Pennsylvania

1. Does not have any specific law for prepaid dental plans.
2. Has a new regulation that covers dental capitation as part of well-developed PPO law.
3. Requires review of proposed plan.
4. Requires capital surplus fund of $50,000 excess above normal liabilities for an insurance company accident and health insurance.
5. Insurance commission reserves the right to reduce capital requirement on a case by case basis. May waive it if dental capitation plan is sound.

Applicable Statutes: Pennsylvania Bulletin, vol. 17, Saturday March 7, 1987, Penn. Statutes Chapter 40, Section 764A, P.L. 226 #64, P.S. 40–364–1551.

Rhode Island

1. Does not have specific legislation for prepaid dental plans.
2. Considers any single-service HMO-type capitation program to be illegal.
3. First HMO started by virtue of a special act of general assembly and set precedent for current law. It is possible that similar thing could be done for dental plans.

Applicable Statutes: Title 27 Chapter 41, General Laws of Rhode Island.

South Carolina

1. Considers dental capitation a line of accident and health insurance.
2. Must have a valid license to offer accident and health insurance.
3. Must submit to an extensive review by the insurance office.
4. Requires an administrator's license to operate any other type of prepaid plan including those modeled after PPOs.
5. Administrator's license requires application with fee of $100.
6. Requires administrator's bond of not less than $50,000.
7. Requires biographical profile of applicant.

Applicable Statutes: South Carolina Insurance Bulletins #80–2, Public Act #133 of 1985.

South Dakota

1. As far as the insurance office is aware, no one has attempted dental capitation in this state.
2. They have no guidelines for regulating it, but are sure that it does not qualify under the HMO Act.
3. They agree that a plan which assumed no risk, like the PPO model, would probably not have to be regulated.
4. Wishes to examine the merits of each plan on an individual basis.

Applicable Statutes: None.

Tennessee

1. Has a special law that allows a Delta plan to operate prepaid capitation plans as well.
2. Others can attempt to qualify under that law if they wish.
3. Requires $75,000 reserve or 55% of gross annual premiums.
4. Requires cash account equal to projected expenses for six months or $2,500, whichever is greater.
5. Requires approval from Tennessee Dental Association.

6. Requires 51% participation of all of the dentists in a given county.
7. Requires 25% participation of all dentists in the state.

Applicable Statutes: TCA 56–30–101.

Texas

1. Regulates prepaid dental plans under the HMO Act as a single-service HMO.
2. Has application procedure with an initial fee of $250 dollars and then an annual reporting fee of $100.
3. Requires a fidelity bond of $100,000.
4. Requires initial surplus assets of $50,000 for Texas residents, and $150,000 for out-of-state owners.
5. Surety deposit of $100,000 plus 4% of each year's gross premiums, until able to qualify for a waiver of this requirement.

Applicable Statutes: HMO Act of Texas Article 20 of the Insurance Code.

Utah

1. Considers prepaid dental plans "Limited Health Plans."
2. Application with fee of $250.
3. Requires a surety bond of $100,000.
4. Requires an initial surplus capital fund of $10,000 to $250,000, depending on anticipated enrollment.
5. Considers PPO-type plans to be a part of this law, but will be more lenient in regulation.

Applicable Statutes: Utah Statutes 31A–8–101 (7) (a).

Vermont

1. Has no legislation.
2. Has not been challenged.
3. Some in office of insurance commission want to regulate; some do not.

4. Wants to examine all plans.
5. Does not regulate discount PPO plans.
6. If governable, it will be under the statute below.

Applicable Statutes: Vermont Statutes Annotated Title 8, 3301, Section 8.

Virginia

1. Has well-defined law for establishing prepaid dental plans.
2. Has application with a $500 fee for filing.
3. Recommends preapplication review by commissioner.
4. Requires financial statement but does not specify amounts for surety and corporate reserves.

Applicable Statutes: Code of Virginia 38.2–4500, 38.2–4208.

Washington

1. Has separate laws dealing with prepaid dental organizations.
2. Has extensive application process with fee of $100.
3. Requires copies of every aspect of operation be filed for scrutiny by the insurance office.
4. Requires surety bond for licensing.
5. Does not regulate PPOs but will require investigation process.

Applicable Statutes: Revised Code F Washington, Chapters 48.44 and 48.46.

West Virginia

1. Does not have specific legislation for prepaid dental plans.
2. Is not currently regulating these types of plans.
3. Has examined prepaid legal plans, and has determined that they are not insurance and therefore is not regulating them either.
4. Has HMO law but dental services are not mentioned.

Applicable Statutes: Chapter 33, Article 25a Insurance Code of West Virginia.

Wisconsin

1. Considers a capitation plan a "Limited Service Health Organization."
2. Has licensing legislation.
3. Has complex licensing rules, and requires a complete package before licensing can be accomplished.

Applicable Statutes: 85–86 Wisconsin Statutes, Chapter 609, also see Chapters 601 and 646.

Wyoming

1. In 1960, Attorney General of Wyoming declared that prepaid dental plans were not insurance and therefore did not have to be regulated.
2. In 1985, Legislature passed an HMO law that in essence reverses that decision.
3. Since law is so new, no companies have attempted to qualify under it.
4. Insurance commission requests that laws be read and then proposal sent to insurance commission for review.

Applicable Statutes: Wyoming Insurance Code Chapter 22 and Chapter 34.

SECTION II

Establishing a Capitation Plan

Chapter 5 Applying for a Capitation License

If DMI Plans wishes to offer dental capitation plans as part of its product, it will most likely be required to obtain a license from the state in which it intends to operate. Because of the assumption of risk, most states consider it insurance. Some states have passed separate legislation dealing specifically with dental capitation. In others, the insurance commissions have interpreted parts of existing legislation that specifically deals with medical HMOs as pertinent to dental capitation. There are still some states that do not regulate these types of programs at all, but if we look at the future, it appears as though all programs will eventually be required to submit to some sort of licensing review. It would be wise to consider this reality before beginning your operation so that when the time comes it will be easier to adjust. Therefore, let's take a look at some of the kinds of things that will be considered by the insurance offices when they evaluate your situation for possible licensure.

For the purposes of explanation, we have chosen the laws of the state of Michigan to serve as our example. Michigan was chosen because of familiarity, and because it has one of the more complicated systems. Michigan can be called an in-between state, because its philosophy regarding prepaid dental plans is not yet clearly defined. Michigan has no specific law covering dental capitation. Instead, it has interpreted a section of its HMO law to apply to these programs. While Michigan has no specific law, it does have a strict set of guidelines which should provide fairly good examples of the various types of things required by other states as well. Perhaps years of union participation in this type of plan has dictated a greater variety of rules. The irony is that in the state of Michigan, at the time of this writing, there is only one licensed prepaid capitation plan. That is not to say that there are not others operating, but they have chosen not to obtain a license. The air surrounding the prepaid concept is filled with controversy. It is conceivable that someone may challenge the legality of this type of regulation without specific legislation.

Certainly there is an immense gray area with regard to the hard-and-fast rules of this game, and there seems to be some legal precedent for the controversy. In the late 1930s the U.S Circuit Court of Appeals upheld a lower court decision in *The District of Columbia Insurance Commission* v. *The Group Health Association of Washington D.C.* that stated that just because the HMO assumed risks, it need not be considered in the business of insurance, and the guarantee to provide service for a prenegotiated amount does not constitute an insurance function, and therefore does not fall under the auspices of the insurance commission. This dichotomy of thought still exists within individual state insurance offices today. The question is, that in light of all of the new legislation, do you want to be the one who tests it in court? That could cost more than you could ever hope of making in this business! But, if you have the money, you could go down in the annals of litigation history—if you need that sort of thing. So for now, check with the charts in the preceding chapter to determine what is required in your state. Does it have a defined law, or does it rely on other legislation and attempt to make rules based on it? Then contact the insurance commission for an application and a copy of the appropriate laws. Remember, the following outline provides a good sampling of the types of things that will be required in order to obtain a license or certificate of authority from just about any state, either currently or some time in the future.

Enabling Legislation

There have been attempts to pass a dental capitation law in the state of Michigan, but as of the date of this writing those attempts have been unsuccessful. The insurance commission uses Chapter 333, Article 17, Part 21042 of the Michigan Public Health Act as its enabling legislation. Check with the preceding chapter to see what the enabling legislation is in your state. That part of the Michigan act reads as follows:

> 333.21042. Health care delivery and financing systems failing to meet requirements of this part: operation, licensing, and regulations.
>
> Sec. 21042. A person proposing to operate a system of health care delivery and financing which is to be offered to individuals whether or not as members of groups in exchange for a fixed payment and organized so that providers and the organization are in some part at risk for the cost of services in a manner similar to a health maintenance organization, but fails to meet the requirements set forth part in this part, may operate such a system if the department and insurance bureau find that the proposed operation will benefit persons who will be served by it. The operation shall be licensed and regulated in the same manner as a Health Maintenance Organization under this part, including the filing of periodic reports except to the extent that the department and

insurance bureau, with the advice of the advisory commission, agree that the regulation is inappropriate to the system of health care delivery and financing. A person operating a system of health care delivery and financing pursuant to this section shall not advertise or solicit in any way identify itself in a manner implying to the public that it is a health maintenance organization.

What they are saying here is, "If you ain't an HMO, then you are something else. And if you're something else, we want to regulate you!" Other states have even more direct wording, but the idea is the same. So, if you are operating some sort of prepaid plan in the state of Michigan, and the insurance commission finds out about it, they will send you a letter asking you to file the appropriate application. They call that a Notice of Opportunity to Show Compliance, or an "NOSC." You may then make the necessary application, or send a letter explaining why your particular plan should not be considered licensable under this part of the Public Health Act.

What they are going to look at predominantly is the assumption of risk. If you are going to collect money in advance and assume the risk for the cost of services delivered later, you will be required to be licensed. If it seems we are belaboring this point, it is for good reason. Dental capitation plans, whether they are delivered directly out of the office or through an intermediary company, assume risk and therefore must be licensed. If you decide not to comply with these rules, you will be given a notice and the opportunity to plead your case directly to the staff of the insurance commission. If they decide against you and you are still intent on operating without the license, the insurance commission may ask the attorney general to prosecute you. The court may issue an order for you to stop your activities, and, in Michigan, you may be in for a fine of $5,000 if you have received any income from your activities. The penalties in other states may be more harsh.

This part of the Public Health Act pretty much sets the rules for offering dental capitation plans, but it may not be all that bad. This section also implies that you may be able to offer a modified plan—one which does not require licensing—by simply writing a letter. We will talk about how to do this later in this book.

For now, let's assume that DMI Plans is bent on offering dental capitation plans as its product and proceed with our discussion of applying for a license. Let's look at some general things from the act and the insurance commission rules regarding HMO/dental capitation plans.

Money in General

The first thing to consider, as always, is money. Just to have your application read in the state of Michigan, it will cost you a $1,000 application fee. In the state of Florida, it is $225. In Arizona, it is only $25, along with a $100 examiner's deposit, which is refundable if your company ceases operation. Why such a big discrepancy? No one knows or is willing to say. Some speculate that some states have better lobbyists whose interests have leaned towards inhibiting competition for the larger indemnifying insurers. Who knows?

Let's stay on the topic of money for a minute. It reflects on a familiar theme: the assumption of risk. If you are taking money in advance for services not yet delivered, the insurance commission wants to be sure you will remain financially viable so that you can deliver the services. According to the Michigan Public Health Act, an HMO must deposit $100,000 into a federally chartered financial institution under an acceptable trust indenture as a surety against insolvency. For an HMO, the deposit can be in cash or securities. For a dental capitation company, the deposit shall be $10,000 to $50,000, depending upon the decision of the insurance commission upon review of your application. They are not sure and intend to make their judgment when they receive all of the facts. This is a typical example of one of those "in-between states." In Arizona, the amount of this surety bond is set expressly in their act. It is based on a sliding scale set on the number of enrollees with whom the company contracts. For 5,000 or fewer members, this deposit is $25,000. It jumps to $30,000 when there are 7,500 members. It runs all the way to $200,000 for 40,000 or more members. In addition, the state of Arizona requires a fidelity bond of $50,000 for each person named to the board of directors of the company. Florida requires no such surety deposit to operate a dental prepaid system.

Also, Michigan requires an organization considering dental capitation plans to maintain a certain working capital fund. They are, however, unable to say just how much that should be. To operate a medical HMO in Michigan, a surety deposit of $100,000 is required and the entity must maintain a working capital fund of at least $250,000. For a dental capitation plan, the surety deposit necessary will be reduced to somewhere between $10,000 and $50,000. Presumably the working capital fund will be reduced as well.

Michigan has an additional requirement in its prepaid law that further demonstrates the principle that money rules. In addition to the previously mentioned funds, a capitation company must keep 5% of its income received from premiums in a fund held by a chartered financial institution. Also they have a clause that stipulates how much net worth a company must be able to demonstrate after a five-year period. If the capitation company does not obtain the determined level, their license may be revoked. Florida has no such percentage of premium requirement nor does it say how much net worth a company must have after a certain time. Arizona also does not dictate growth, nor does it require additional deposits other than the 2% for financial reserve.

The rules in Michigan serve to demonstrate some key points to developing your own dental capitation plans. They are the direct children of the HMOs; they are then ultimately governed by the HMO Act of 1973. The dominating factor when discussing such entities is the assumption of risk. The federal law and the subsequent state laws outline certain specifics regarding financial solvency to insure that the risk is adequately protected. Some states are just tougher than others! Check it out before you start. The table from the preceding chapter that shows which laws are applicable in your state should help. If you do not think you can handle the financial limitations, don't waste your time. If you are a solo or small group practice in the state of Michigan, and you think you want to offer dental capitation plans out of your office, forget it! If you are in Florida, it may be likely that you could succeed. We should restate the importance of reading the current laws and asking pertinent questions to the insurance commissioners. These laws and enforcement policies are changing constantly. By the time this goes to press, even Michigan may have more definitive policies.

For the solo practitioner, that first bombshell regarding basic finances may have been enough to flatten your plans about offering dental capitation plans directly out of your small office. However, a way for offering some sort of plan still exists. (We'll discuss it in Section III of this book.) For those of you who think you may have enough horsepower to gather your friends together and form a capitation company, or those considering developing an IPA to handle plans others are developing, or those with small group practices and multiple office groups with sufficient resources to handle the financial requirements, let's continue our discussion of obtaining a license to offer capitation plans. Dental capitation will be one of the major forces on the horizon of the industry for a long time to come and as the trend for solos to merge into groups continues, it is realistic that plans could be delivered directly out of an office if it is large enough.

Querying the Commission

Generally speaking, DMI Plans will have to furnish statements that reflect the following:

1. Organizational structure
2. Service area
3. Type and location of facilities to be utilized
4. Projected population to be served and the number of prospective enrollees
5. Description of marketing concepts and proposed procedures.
6. Estimated cost for establishment and for first-year operation
7. Proposed sources of financing for the organization, including estimated amounts
8. Services to be provided

At this point, it might be a good idea to think seriously about each of these eight items, and design a short protocol that describes your—and the rest of your group's—thoughts about them. Write it up in some sort of brief format that clearly states what it is that you intend to do specifically in regard to each of these concepts. Send it to the insurance commissioner and ask him what he thinks your possibilities are for acceptance. Many of the decisions about licensing are made on a discretionary basis by the commissioner. If you approach the project properly and personally, giving him as much information as possible, you may find your quest easier to obtain. You might even consider a meeting between your group, your attorney, and the commissioner to informally discuss your plans. You may even find it helpful to establish your proposed corporate bylaws in advance of this initial meeting. You will have to do it eventually anyway, and by doing it in advance you will be able to clearly outline some of your goals and needs going in. In this regard, you may find it helpful to consult the *Nichols Cyclopedia of Legal Forms Annotated, Volume 7A.* It presents a concise guide to forming a medical HMO, complete with corporate bylaws, contract outlines, and formats for various other corporate structures. By making the necessary changes and deletions to convert the medical format to dental format, you may find it to be an invaluable shortcut in creating your new entity. *Nichols Cyclopedia of Legal Forms* can be found at most law libraries. Remember to do your homework with regard to the eight items, so that your first impression is favorable. Remember too, it is human nature—and the particular nature of bureaucratic officials—to tell you all of the reasons why you can't do something. Remain positive and concentrate on how you can!

The purpose of the preliminary proposal is twofold. First, it will help to crystallize in your mind, and the mind of your associates, what it is that you intend to do. Secondly, it should give you an idea of how practical it will be before you plunge in so to speak. Filing a proper application requires the use of lawyers, accountants, research companies, and possibly even actuarial statisticians. That can be quite costly. Indeed, it could cost ten times the application fee. Compare your optimistic expectations to the initial reaction to your plan. If after examination of your preliminary proposal, you feel the chances are good that you will be able to succeed, then go for it!

The best way to start is to obtain a copy of the governing legislation particular to your state and read it. Then read a copy of the rules and regulations established by your individual insurance office. Then, if they offer one, and Michigan does, read a copy of the guidelines for applying, noticing the particular nuances each regulatory commission may have. Michigan even describes the type of stationery you should use in addition to the type of binder it should have. Take each portion of the application and concentrate on it specifically, writing as good a description of your plans as possible. Be specific. Be professional. Put forth a proposal that will shed the light of credibility upon your project.

General Licensing Guidelines

Each state has variations, but generally they want to make sure that your program is administered properly, and that your business format is sound. Michigan goes so far as to define how your governing body shall be established and mandates that there be a method of electing subscriber representatives to your governing board. They specify that you will have to have a licensed practitioner as medical director on your governing board. This director must not have a direct conflict of interest with regards to the decisions he makes and the benefit of the public and the corporation. The state of Florida requires an investigative background report on each of the partners, stockholders, directors, presidents, chiefs, and other staff members. They will accept a report prepared by a private company engaged in investigating individuals and providing reports and background profiles to prospective employers. If your state requires in-depth personal reporting about corporate officers, you may find one of these services to be an expressway to accomplishing that part of the problem.

Guiding Your Operation

As you examine each part of the application, you will find details that will answer questions you may have regarding the day-to-day operation of your business. You can almost use the application itself as a guide as to how to structure your operation. The Michigan rules mandate:

1. All the activities of the board of directors of your company
2. Which policies must be written
3. Enrollee grievance procedures
4. Communications summaries
5. Marketing and enrollment policies
6. Programs to ensure continuity of treatment for enrollees
7. Contractural arrangements with outside resources required to complement and supplement services available to enrollees.

In addition, they have established other administrative guidelines which include:

1. Rules regarding the frequency of governing board meetings
2. Quorum requirements
3. Record-keeping procedures
4. Meeting proceedings reports
5. Notice of meetings
6. Minutes

They say a capitation company must have a principle location (a physical office) and a name. The capitation company cannot change either of these without prior written approval from the commissioner. It is further required that they notify the commissioner of any transfers of stock which result in one person owning more than 10% of the voting shares of the company. The Michigan rules go on to dictate:

1. Accounting procedures
2. Establishment of a fiscal year
3. Financial and budgetary projections
4. Establishment of a financial plan which
   a. Identifies the means of achieving positive cash flow
   b. Demonstrates an approach to the risk of insolvency
   c. Provides a surety bond issued by an independent bonding company
   d. Provides a reinsurance contract
   e. Provides a sound contract with providers that insures solvency
   f. Identifies a group of potential subscribers
   g. Offers a guaranteed line of credit
   h. Projects fixed developmental costs
   i. Establishes the 5% contingency reserve fund
   j. Provides an appropriate amount of working capital

In addition Michigan rules describe:

1. Methods used to establish rates
2. Methods used to establish co-pays
3. Methods used to establish deductibles
4. How reinsurance contracts will be established and monitored
5. How general liability insurance will be established and monitored, including fire, theft, general liability, and malpractice insurance.

Michigan reserves the right to approve or disapprove:

1. Provider contracts and amendments. It should be noted that the insurance commissioner reserves the right to reject a provider contract at any time, provided he gives 60 days written notice of his intent.

The Michigan rules address other topics such as:

1. How to establish standards for service

2. How to establish staffing guidelines
3. How to establish quality control procedures
4. How to establish utilization review procedures
5. How to establish facility standards
6. How to maintain clinical records
7. Monitoring and reporting of clinical procedures

The Michigan rules provide guidelines for marketing and enrollment methods such as:

1. Description of data used to project enrollment
2. Methodology and assumptions used for enrollment data
3. Outlining the number and kind of marketing people
4. Describing methods used to ensure accountability of enrollment representatives
5. Approval of all proposed promotional, advertising, and informational materials
6. Description of enrollment procedures including application forms and processing steps
7. Monitoring and approval of any sales arrangements the company may involve itself in

Formatting Additional Concepts

This outline of the procedures involved in obtaining a capitation license in the state of Michigan serves two purposes. First of all, it demonstrates the kinds of things anyone who is considering starting and operating a dental capitation plan should incorporate into his stratagem. Secondly, it should hint at a common theme which will make the development of everything hich follows easier. The threads that form the fabric of the HMO Act weave themselves through every document involved with the capitation concept. Every clause in a provider contract can be traced back through the act, into the state act, into the rules for operation sanctioned by the commissions, into the application, through the promotional literature, through the plan proposals, into the subscriber contracts, and back again to the original contract. It is this circular cycling of ideas (figure 2), that hangs like a wreath on the door to successful development of a capitation plan. To develop any aspect of a contract, or a campaign, or even corporate bylaws, one needs only to thread each fiber through its appropriate loop and into its proper place.

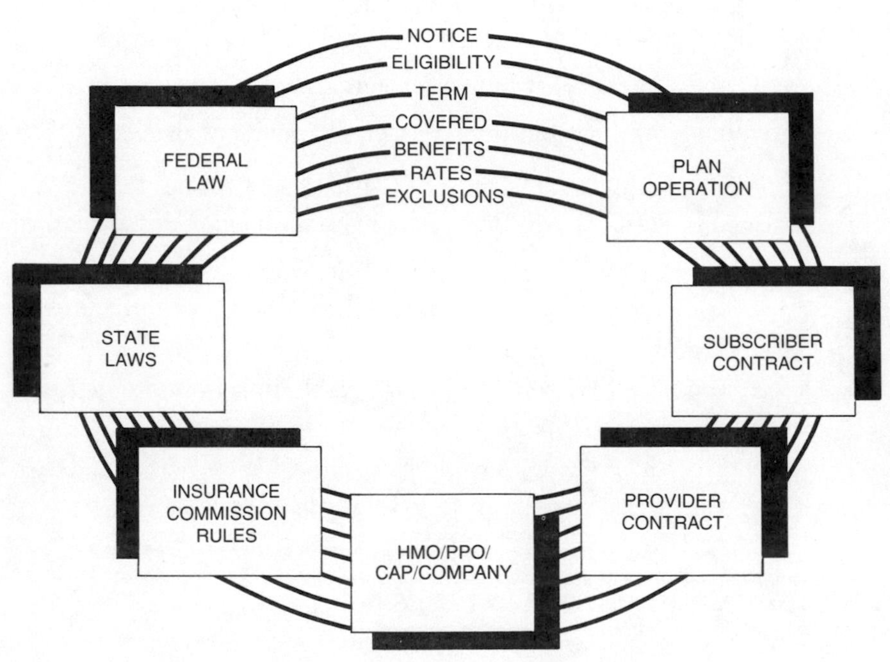

Chapter 6 Provider Relations

We have said that there are four major areas of concern when considering starting prepaid dental plans. They are legality, marketing strategy, subscriber relations, and provider relations. DMI Plans cannot directly deliver dental services. Keep that principle in mind when formulating your ideas about subscriber contracts. You will want a clause in every contract, and even in your plan proposals, that specifically addresses this principle. DMI Plans will want it known that they are only promising to use their best efforts to obtain licensed providers to deliver specific health care services to members of the plan under predetermined guidelines. DMI Plans obviously cannot drill and fill itself. Therefore, it must have strong relations with providers to deliver those services. It will require bilateral contracts which will define both the roles of the providers and DMI Plans exactly.

Soliciting Providers

The first step to provider relations is to find some provider to relate to. If you are a multiple office group with enough providers to handle the geographic and pretargeted market segment, then don't worry about this. All you will need is a contract between you and DMI Plans to make it official. However, you may see the need to incorporate more providers into the plan in order to handle a specific large group or simply to fulfill your original marketing intentions. Indeed, you may find it necessary to show the commissioner of insurance a suitable number of willing providers before you are ever granted a license.

To do that, you will need to define some guidelines you will use to determine those practitioners who may qualify as providers for your plan. Unfortunately, some dentists are not candidates for participation in dental capitation plans. The HMO Act of 1973 contains some restrictions that may make it difficult for a small-time operator to function in a state that interprets dental HMO laws in the same manner as medical HMOs. For example, the HMO Act stipulates that HMOs must provide 24-hour emergency service. A solo practitioner in a rural area, who has one or two chairs, may not be able to handle that requirement. You may find it difficult to compete unless you are able to offer some sort of expanded hours. Once again, it may be impractical for the solo practitioner to handle the necessary expansion in staff and hours to accommodate his marketing plans. In contrast, a small group with one or two practitioners and some extra chair time on their hands may be quite capable of handling the load. It depends a bit on what DMI Plans intends to do. If it is content to offer only small plans to small groups in limited geographic areas, then it may be quite possible that a small solo practitioner could handle the additional load with ease. The risky part with capitation plans is that they work better when their principles are applied to larger volumes ofpatients. The financial requirements of licensing alone may bankrupt the company before it ever gets started if there is not sufficient volume to offset them within a couple of years of operation.

You can see that you will have to establish a criterion for acceptance into the plan, and develop some sort of screening application to go along with your letter of solicitation. If you have been practicing dentistry in this country in the last few years, no doubt you have already received a letter of this type in the mail. Their purpose is to try to solicit your participation in a particular dental plan. They are all slightly different, but essentially they read something like this:

> Dear Doctor,
>
> DMI Plans is an internationally recognized leader in dental health care programs serving a wide range of private employer/employee groups as well as a number of popular associations. We are currently seeking practitioners to participate in our programs in your area.
>
> You will find our plans to be a valuable adjunct to the way in which you have delivered high quality dental services. They promise to provide you the opportunity to continue to serve a wide cross section of new patients.
>
> Sound interesting? If you think you would like to join a rapidly expanding team of health care professionals who are enjoying the increase in patient loads our plans provide, please fill out and return the questionnaire enclosed, and one of our representatives will contact you soon.
>
> We are looking forward to having you on our team, and wish you continued success in the future.
>
> Sincerely,
>
> DMI Plans

OK—this one lays it on a little thick, but you get the point. If you perceive the necessity of involving other practitioners in your program, you will need a solicitation device similar to this one. Naturally, the best solicitation is word of mouth. If you have friends who you think may be interested in helping you to deliver services under your capitation plan, by all means ask them! The core of most prepaid plans is made up of individuals who share a common interest, and who may have worked together before. Conceivably, you are considering this entire project already because you have a group of providers who can deliver the services out of their offices. If so, you won't need the solicitation letter; you can move on.

Office Questionnaire

The next item to consider under the category of provider relations is an office questionnaire. The very core of capitation plans is the closed panel. You simply do not want every practitioner in the plan. It is a tightrope of sorts. You must have enough practitioners to build your credibility, both with prospective clients and the licensing officials, but at the same time, you must be sure that each provider in the system shares in the number of patients to the extent the participation in the plan works out to be profitable for them. And to emphasize, if you require licensing for your project, you may find that the commissioner will want to have viable proof that you will have sufficient providers to make it work.

The questionnaire should begin with the standard name, rank, and serial number sort of information. Name, location, telephone number, major cross streets, and the year the practice was founded should be included in the first part of the form. A schedule should follow that will outline the approximate hours the office is open. It should have a place for the respondent to indicate what type of practice it is—solo, group, partnership, corporation, etc. It should have a space to indicate whether any specialists work out of the office who would be willing to contribute to the plan. The form should provide for the names of all of the practitioners working under the general name of the practice. It should list all of the auxiliary personnel, including assistants, hygienists, office and administrative personnel, and the approximate number of hours they work each week. The total number of operatories is important, and the form should specify how many chairs are used for general dentistry, and how many for hygiene. There should be an indication of the number of x-ray units available, and whether or not there are any laboratory facilities available on the premises. In addition, you will want to know if emergency treatment is currently available and under what method it is offered. It might be helpful to know what type of recall system the office uses, and if any other policies and programs are used to monitor the internal functioning of the office. Is there some form of quality assessment procedure, or peer review function? It may be helpful to know if any patient education programs are in effect, and how they are administered. Group offices and satellites are important as well. If you do not wish to make your own form for gathering this information or are uncomfortable deciding which practitioners to admit into the program, you can get a questionnaire and a list of acceptable criteria from the American Academy of Dental Group Practice. They have an Accreditation Program that could be helpful. This is how Blue Cross/Blue Shield's Dental Network of America makes its decisions.

Choosing Providers

Once you have collected the information, you will have a basis to decide which offices you would like to have in your group. In some cases the decision may be difficult, and you may want to keep an office in mind as an alternate for the future if it becomes necessary. In other cases, you may find that because of location and willingness of providers to participate, the decision is not as critical. You may have to use a combination of smaller offices in the same general location to handle the program if there are no larger groups available.

You may run into a pitfall here. In some states the various dental organizations are attempting to lobby for legislation mandating "freedom of choice." The intent is that no dentist be prevented from becoming a provider in any program as long as he was willing to abide by the terms of the provider contract. Check to see if your state has any such legislation, but don't worry about it too much. It is unlikely that anyone will challenge you,but if you have to let someone in who is not right for the program in one way or another, it really won't matter much. Patients may not sign up for his office if he is too bad. If not he does not make any money, he will want to drop out himself. Be sure to set up an office in his immediate area which can handle the plan so that patients have somewhere to go in the event there are problems. That in itself may be a deterrent, but if not, talk to him. Point out how his credibility will be affected even more than yours by his failure to operate efficiently under the plan. The risk to you of a provider invoking a freedom of choice law on you is minimal. At the very least, he may be able to deliver some services to your clients. So let him.

Provider Contracts

Once you have made the decision about which offices to accept into the plan, you will then have to have the signatures of the corporate officers on a specialized provider contract. Before we discuss provider contracts, it is important to remember that each state has guidelines and specific forms necessary to make the contract valid. It is mandatory that you make a trip to the attorney to assure that your contract is valid for your particular area. In addition, remember that any contracts used in the prepaid dental business should carry the same elemental threads that pass through the HMO Act of 1973, the subsequent state statutes, the rules and regulations of the insurance office, and any additional statutes that may be germane to your plan.

Opening

Most contracts begin by identifying the parties involved in the agreement, and specifying the date that it becomes effective. Ours might read as follows:

> THIS AGREEMENT is entered into this ___ day of ______ ,19 __ , by and between Dental Maintenance International (hereinafter referred to as "DMI Plans"), a duly authorized corporation, licensed to do business as a for-profit corporation and ________ DDS, and __________ DDS, Individually and d/b/a ____________________ sole proprietorship, a partnership, or corporation, all of whom are licensed to practice dentistry (hereinafter referred to as the "Dentists," whether one or more).

Recitals

The next part of the agreement is some statement of pertinent facts. Some refer to it as a recital of events that have bearing on the agreement which follows. Ours might say something like this:

Witnesseth:

WHEREAS, DMI Plans is a licensed corporation, providing various groups and associations with dental care for their members under the following guidelines, and said services are provided on a closed panel basis; and

WHEREAS, DMI Plans has established various contracts with various groups, and has agreed to provide group members with dental services as defined herein for periodic prepayment of fees; and

WHEREAS, it is understood that the contracts mentioned above may from time to time be changed, and that each contract may contain individual clauses that may vary, and that additional contracts may be added from time to time, and that the Dentist may be responsible for provisions of those contracts as well, subject to the terms and conditions set forth under this contract; and

WHEREAS, the Dentist represents and warrants that the Dentist is duly licensed to provide dental services and is certified by the board of examiners, and that the Dentist is desirous of providing services for DMI Plans, under the terms defined herein; and

WHEREAS, DMI Plans wishes to contract with said Dentist to provide services to members of groups and associations with whom it has contracted;

NOW, THEREFORE, the parties do mutually covenant and agree as follows:

Definitions

Most provider contracts then turn their attention to a list of definitions. Each varies as to which terms it cares to list in this section and the extent to which it defines them. A sample of a few of the terms our contract might use follows:

Definitions of Certain Terms Used Herein

1. Member. (Could be subscriber, enrollee, participant, or patient.) A person who is actually enrolled in the DMI Plan and is eligible to receive services as provided herein under one of the groups or organizations under contract with DMI Plans. The term "Member" or "Members" as used in this agreement shall be deemed to include all eligible dependents of a member as defined herein.

2. Dependents. The member's lawful spouse and unmarried children to age nineteen (19) or any unmarried children to age twenty three (23) who attend an accredited institution on a full-time basis and are dependent wholly on the member for their support.

3. Dentist. Any dental care provider duly licensed to provide services and any auxiliary personnel practicing within the scope of said license, including hygienists, assistants, technicians, or shareholders of the corporation, as well as its principals, agents, or employees.

4. Dental Review Panel. A group of licensed dental care practitioners selected annually by the Board of Directors of DMI Plans to review the manners, operations, costs, and necessity of the services provided by the Dentist.

Length Of Contract

We could include other definitions in this part of the contract. Indeed, many do. Some include in this section wording regarding upcoming paragraphs dealing with the methods of compensation to the dentist, and the way in which the capitation company will take its percentage of the money the dentist gets. Let's let this serve for now and move on to the next common section of the provider contract, the term of the agreement. Some provider contracts do not specify a definite length that the contract will remain in effect. This may be a good method for setting up your plan, since it eliminates the necessity of having to set up another signing each time the contract comes due. Wording for this clause may be something like this:

Duration of Agreement. This agreement shall continue until terminated by the Dentist upon ninety (90) days prior written notice to DMI Plans or terminated by DMI Plans upon ninety (90) days written notice to the Dentist.

Another way of handling the renewal problem is to specify the exact term of the agreement and then include an automatic renewal clause at this point:

Term. This agreement shall be in effect as of the date of execution hereof and shall remain in effect for a period of one (1) year, unless terminated by either party upon thirty (30) days notice in writing to the other party. Further, this agreement shall automatically renew each and every year hereafter, for a period of one (1) year upon the same terms and conditions.

An important point to consider here is the length of time necessary to terminate the contract. If you are in the fortunate position of having potential providers clamoring for the chance to join the program, then a short time such as thirty days might be acceptable. But, if you perceive that it might be difficult to find a provider to accept your patients or contractees, as might be true in a rural area, then perhaps it would be wise to increase the length of time necessary to effect a termination in order to give yourself ample time to locate another provider. It works both ways, though. If you need to boot a guy for abuses in the program, it will take longer. Fortunately, patients are not dumb. They will cease to seek services from a bad practitioner, no matter what financial arrangements exist, and that in itself will buy you some time.

One final item regarding term of the contract. The threads of logic that originate in the law must flow consistently through each instrument used in dental prepaid contracting. In a similar manner, the methods used to operate the plan on a day-to-day basis must be traceable to those instrumnts as well. Variable points negotiated with subscribers must be supported by contracts with providers. If you intend to offer one-year contracts with subscribers, then one year contracts with providers will be adequate. If, however, you foresee the possibility that you may want to offer longer contracts with subscribers (there are some valid arguments for this) then you should make sure that your provider contracts match. You will want to avoid the development of a situation in which your provider contracts expire before your subscriber contracts do, or you will suddenly be faced with having to find other providers to service your clients.

Who Does What—and Malpractice

Next, our contract should be sure to point out the differences between the dentist and the capitation company. DMI Plans does not want to assume any liability that may arise out of the actual delivery of the services by the dentist. It may be advisable to specify how much malpractice insurance the individual dentist must carry, and that he assuredly must carry it! Additionally, this might be a good place to include any other rules for the dentist that might be included in the regulations of your particular state. This part might go something like this:

Independent Relationships. It is specifically agreed and understood that in performing the services herein described, the Dentist is acting as an independent contractor and not as an agent or employee of DMI Plans. The Dentist shall maintain the dentist-patient relationship with the members DMI Plans has contracted with, and shall be solely responsible to the patient for the dental advice and treatment. It is expressly agreed that neither the groups or organizations contracted with, or DMI Plans shall have dominion or control over the Dentist's practice or procedures, or the Dentist's personnel or facilities. The Dentist hereby agrees to hold harmless, defend, and indemnify DMI Plans and any of its contracting groups and organizations, their board of directors, officers, employees, agents, or administrators from any claims, suits, demands, actions, etc., that may arise out of any alleged malpractice or negligent act or omission to act, caused or alleged to have been caused by the Dentist or any of his agents, employees, consultants, associates, owners, or partners in the performance or omission of any professional duty assumed by dentist hereunder.

Malpractice Insurance. The Dentist shall provide evidence of malpractice insurance coverage of one million dollars ($1,000,000) per occurrence through the entire term of this contract. The Dentist shall provide DMI Plans with a copy of an endorsement that names DMI Plans as as "Additional Insured" within forty-five (45) days of the execution of this agreement. The Dentist shall notify DMI Plans within ten (10) days of cancellation of this coverage.

With the increased numbers of litigations leveled at dentists, lawyers are drawing their sights on everyone who may be connected with a possible malpractice claim in even the most remote way. If your organization is anything other than an incorporated entity, you may have an increased exposure to a malpractice action. You may be insulated a bit if you are incorporated, but nonetheless, you will no doubt be forced to hire an attorney to defend you if you are named in a malpractice suit against a dentist in your system, or against yourself, if you are a provider, since the prepaid entity is a separate entity. Win or lose, this will cost you money. It may be wise to add another paragraph to your provider contract to help offset these potential costs. Say something like the following:

Should DMI Plans be forced to defend itself in any lawsuit, claim, demand, or action for any malpractice or negligence, on the part of the

> Dentist, the Dentist agrees to pay any liabilities, attorneys fees, court costs, or other expenses, associated with said defense.

Next, we will want to specify to the dentist that he must serve the clients we send him. He must know that it is his responsibility to treat any and all patients that we have contracted with so that we are not left assuming all of the risk instead of him—which is the underlying principle of capitation. We should have in our provider contract a paragraph that reads something like this:

> The Dentist agrees to render all dental services set forth in the various contracts between DMI Plans and groups or organizations, to each Member of said group or organization who may present to his office.

DMI Plans will want to preserve its options for future business, and will want the dentist to know that he may have to accept patients from additional groups in the future. We may want to add wording such as this:

> It is further understood that DMI Plans may enter into contracts with new groups or organizations during the term of this contract and that the Dentist may be responsible for the delivery of services as provided herein, subject to the terms and conditions of this agreement.

Because dental plans are changing about as fast as the ability of creative minds to think them up, you might want to set up provisions for the possibility that you may have to change your basic contract from time to time in order to offer new products and remain competitive. If you anticipate the need for a variety of contracts and even a variety of fee schedules, you may want to give the provider the opportunity to participate on a contract-to-contract basis. Admittedly, this may create extra paperwork and increased headaches, but it may be necessary if DMI Plans wants to remain flexible in a rapidly changing economic marketplace. Try this wording:

> The Dentist must notify DMI Plans within seven (7) days that it does not wish to participate in a particular DMI Plans contract. If written notification is not received by DMI Plans within the allocated time period, Dentist shall be deemed to have agreed to participate. Such refusal to participate in a particular contract does not in any way affect the Dentist's participation with other previously existing contracts. Refusal to participate in three (3) contracts in any calendar year shall

constitute a breach of this contract, and may be grounds for termination of the agreement.

Providers and Members

Section 1301, subsection B, paragraph 4 of the Health Maintenance Act of 1973 states that the services be available to members promptly, and delivered in a manner which assures continuity. Additionally, it specifies that emergency services be accessible twenty four hours a day, seven days a week. There is presumably some leeway with regard to supplemental services such as dental services, and assuredly some differences between dentists and patients as to what constitutes an emergency, but basically dental capitation plans should follow similar guidelines as part of the burden of assuming the risk. Therefore we should add some words to our provider contract outlining how the dentist will deliver services to insure that our member contracts are properly covered.

It is agreed that the Dentist shall provide services during his normal working hours and in addition the Dentist agrees to provide services during additional hours as may be deemed necessary by DMI Plans in order to keep appointment schedules on a reasonable basis in accordance with DMI Plans contracts with groups or organizations. Emergency care will be available as soon as possible and in priority to all other appointments. The Dentist agrees that his office will be covered for emergencies during vacations and other periods his office might normally be closed. Non-emergency services shall be given not more than three (3) weeks after the time requested by the participant.

The three-week appointment rule is important. Remember, establishing credibility is of paramount concern. If patients have to wait forever to be seen by one of your dentists, they will begin to have doubts about your program. The result of this is that they may fail to re-sign your contract in subsequent years when the profts of individual providers in the plan will begin to increase. That will bruise credibility fast. Since providers are paid in advance under capitation plans and in essence make more if they do not have to deliver services or if they can postpone delivering them, there might be a temptation to put off appointments while still enjoying that monthly capitation premium. This might be particularly true with supplemental services like orthodontics, or replacing noncritical missing teeth. The three-week rule gives you some control. On the down side though, it selects against the smaller office. It is another reason why choosing a small office to provide services for your plan in an area where you may have a lot of subscribers may not be a good idea. You don't want the dentist so swamped that he can not deliver services within a reasonable time even if he tries.

While we're on the subject of delivering services to our clients, it might be wise to address another consideration. The capitation concept labors with one underlying economic assumption. When a new group of subscribers joins the program, invariably their initial utilization of the program will be high. High utilization means the dentists deliver a greater number of services while their monthly share of the capitation premium remains the same. It is possible during the first part of any plan that the provider will actually lose some money. However, as time goes on, if the providers in the system have been doing a good job, the necessity of providing services should drop and utilization should begin to decline as well. Now the situation is reversed. The dentist is still receiving that monthly capitation rate, but is no longer delivering services so his profits increase proportionally. This is a strong argument for the concept of preventive dentistry. No doubt Elwood had this in mind when he first proposed the HMO concept to Congress. Get the participants, as a group, to a reasonable level of health, and then all you will have to do is maintain it, and the overall costs will decrease. A good capitation manager, or provider for that matter, knows this and dreams of that ideal situation when all of his subscribers are happily paying their premiums while they float contentedly in a recall system without the need for services. That would be the best of all possible worlds with individuals on both sides of the contracts in medical bliss, but it seldom happens just that way. The idea though, is to strive for the adequate prevention and monitoring and reduce the need to continually provide services. The offshoot from the capitation providers and managers is a satisfied group of clients who readily re-sign their contracts in subsequent years when they may require little treatment.

Unfortunately some providers might view this differently by assuming that if they never see the patients at all they will not have to deliver any services, and they can enjoy the premiums with impunity. Therefore, we should remind them through our provider contract of the basic premise of capitation—success for both providers and subscribers.

> The Dentist shall have during the entire term he is servicing any contract for DMI Plans, an adequate and effective recall system, and any member of a group or organization under contract to DMI Plans who presents for service at the office of the Dentist shall be entered into said recall system and his records adequately maintained.

Specialists and Risk Pools

We must open a can of worms and we might as well open it right now, because we will need to refer to it again later. It is the question of specialty referrals. Traditionally, under the capitation concept the providers assume the risk for all of the treatment needs of the subscribers. If we are talking about a large HMO with access to hospitals and huge staffs that can handle any situation, the problem is for the most part self-negating. When we are talking about the individual dentist delivering services directly out of his office, the problem looms large. Indeed, it has been a source of complaints and rejection of capitation plans by practitioners since their inception.

If a provider is responsible for all of the treatments required by a patient, he must pay for the referral to a specialist if the need arises. One case of severely impacted third molars that must be referred to a specialist could easily wipe out all of the profits made on premiums for several families over an entire year. The dentist has two options: (1) treat the case himself, and incur the risk of possible malpractice in the event something goes wrong, or (2) do not refer the patient at all. This second choice may not be available when pain and dysfunction motivate the patient to seek relief. The problem never solves itself in the case where orthodontic intervention is necessary.

A couple of reasons for the existence of this problem are obvious. First of all, how can specialists in the system share in the capitation premiums? The primary care provider is assuming most of the risk for providing the services to the subscribers. He therefore must receive the lion's share of the premium. There is no group which will not require a cleaning at least once a year. This is a requirement of good dental care, and the standard of treatment in most areas. Conceivably, however, one could imagine a group which may not need a specialty root canal in a given year. How then can the services of an endodontist be capitated? It is even more likely that a group could be envisioned who did not need orthodontics. Indeed, orthodontic emergencies are almost nonexistent.

One way of lessening the burden of speciality referrals is to provide for increased co-pays for those services. Unfortunately, standard co-pays never even approach a fee sufficient to entice a specialist to assume the risk for his services. That brings us to the second reason for the overall problem of specialty referrals: specialists simply do not need to join any provider groups. They have enjoyed a unique position in the hierarchy of dental services for so long that there has never been much of a need for them to participate in any program where a discount of fees is necessary. They have simply not been affected by the increased numbers of practitioners diluting the supply- and-demand equation. At the risk of sounding offensive, they have enjoyed a prima donna position and are resistant to change. Orthodontists have enjoyed this position to an even greater extent because of the tremendous fee associated with their time-consuming service.

Times are changing a bit even for the specialists. The increase in practitioners has meant that a spillover into the specialty fields is inevitable. Some specialty providers have elected to join plans and are paid in a variety of ways. This may be particularly true in an area where there are an abundance of beginning specialists who are eager to see their practices grow at a rate ahead of their incredible start-up costs. The ideal situation for the manager of a capitation company is to find those provider offices who already have specialists on staff and pay them internally. This points once again to the need to seek those larger group practices as providers as opposed to the small solo offices, where an on-staff specialist is unlikely.

If it is impossible to find enough group offices with on-staff specialists (whose services can be used through conventional salary mechanisms instead of the sharing of capitation premiums), the next best thing is to find those specialty providers who are hungry enough to accept your co-pay rates as payment in full for their services. It is important then that they receive enough volume to make it worth their while. If they are attempting to build up a new practice they may benefit by treating increased numbers of satisfied patients, and the referrals of fee-for-service patients that satisfaction may generate. Nonetheless, you will find this to be one of the most frustrating aspects of managing a dental capitation program. It will require your sharpest sales skills.

If you cannot find any specialists who are willing to accept your plan, you may have to sweeten the pot. The easiest way to accomplish this is to raise the co-pays for specialty services. The obvious risk here is that if you raise them too much, you may risk reducing the appeal of the plan to the prospective subscribers. It is difficult to balance oneself on this swaying tightrope. It is especially difficult considering the changes that may be necessary if you are too far off one way or the other. It is sort of like the chicken-and-the-egg conundrum. If you preset speciality co-pays to attract specialists, you may not be able to sign enough subscribers to facilitate the system. If you sell the plan to the subscribers at a given specialty fee, you may find it difficult to solicit specialists if the fee is too low. We'll talk about setting co-pay fees again later. Remember, higher co-pays generally mean lower premiums, and vice versa.

If you are still having problems with the specialist question, you might try establishing some sort of method for the specialists to share in the monthly capitation payments. The difficulty here comes from trying to match a particular practitioner with a particular group of subscribers, and then trying to justify a premium share on the basis of potential use. You may find actuarial statistics to be of value, in an attempt to predict how many members of a particular group will need which services over a given period of time. If you apply those statistics to the group with whom you are contracting, you may be able to guess at an appropriate capitation rate. If you are successful, keep in mind that if you pay the specialists in your program part of the premiums, it will dilute the funds available to pay the generalists. That means higher co-pays, and the cycle starts all over again.

By far the most common method of solving this complex issue is to use a concept called *risk pooling*. As its name implies, under a risk pool plan, the administrator sets aside a percentage of the money collected in the form of premiums to form a payment pool. Individual dental procedures are then assigned a relative value, or a weight, usually referred to as a unit. When a dentist completes a particular procedure, he is credited with the units assigned to that procedure. At the end of a given payment period, the dollars in the pool are divided by the total amount of the units performed by all the providers in the system, and a dollar amount is then assigned each unit. The various providers are paid the amount due them based on the number of units they are credited with. Each plan may be further limited by plan maximums and minimums.

There are about as many variations to this concept as there are dental plans in existence. Some providers are paid exclusively according to the number of units they produce, without the aid of any sharing of the monthly capitation premium. This is the method most frequently employed in the IPA. A dentist may be paid a portion of the capitation premium in addition to his respective unit share. The pool might be used to pay specialists exclusively. The generalists are paid by means of the monthly capitated premiums remaining after deductions to fund the speciality pool. This is frequently the case where risk pools are established to handle orthodontics.

One program in the state of Michigan makes use of another twist to the risk pool concept. This plan assigns unit value to procedures in much the same way other risk pool plans do, but then they pay specialists their usual fee-for-service (with some limitations). Obviously this drains the pool of resources, so they require the referring dentist to reimburse the pool for 43% of the specialist fee. This has resulted in considerable controversy because it places the total risk of providing services on the general dentists and eliminates any risk for the specialists—not a particularly popular idea. It is not far removed from the old practice of the generalist merely paying the specialist bill out of the capitation fees he received when the patient needed additional services. A plan like this lends itself too easily to abuse. The tendency might be to avoid referrals if they will cost additional money.

Risk pools are the most common method of sharing revenue with specialists. They may not be the best, but a superior method may not have yet been found. One that shifts the responsibility for specialty referrals back to the subscribers can be found in some parts of the country. In such a plan, specialty referrals are simply not covered. They are not listed in the table of allowances or in a benefit schedule. If a patient needs the services of a specialist, he must pay for it himself. This is by far the simplest method for dealing with the specialist issue. If you think about it, it is the fairest to all members of the group because subscribers are not contributing dollars for services they themselves may not ever need. Only those who actually need the treatment pay. Sounds great, doesn't it? It really is the best plan and the easiest to manage. One of its drawbacks is that patients will still think specialty services are covered no matter how many times you tell them they aren't. Make sure that it is spelled out in the subscriber contract. Put it into the plan proposal and in any promotional literature that you distribute. But no matter; they will still think the treatments are covered. Another drawback to a plan like this is that without specialty services it becomes very basic. There is nothing wrong with basic, however, especially if you are offering it to those groups who do not have any coverage to begin with. If you are trying to compete with indemnifying plans that cover ninety percent of anything at any office, you will find it difficult to keep the client's interest. So, if you offer it as a basic benefits plan, do all the specialty services you feel comfortable with and try to provide as many treatments as possible to increase your overall credibility and the good faith of your subscribers but back out of the specialty services that you cannot handle.

No matter which type of plan you end up offering or what specialty arrangements you finally make, it is imperative that you define the provisions of the plan clearly in your provider contract (and all of your subsequent contracts and promotional literature) so that it is clear just exactly what you are offering. If DMI Plans decides to make the povider dentist responsible for specialty referrals, its provider contract should specify that in a manner similar to this:

> **Specialty Referral.** In the event a specialist is required for the treatment of any covered services for the Member, the Dentist shall be responsible for making arrangements for the provision of such specialty services. The Dentist shall also be responsible for the payment to the specialist for the charges incurred as a result of the service rendered to

the patient by the specialist, less any applicable co-payment. The Dentist shall not be responsible for payment of any excluded treatments.

It will be in the best interest of DMI Plans to try to sign up as many specialists as possible to (1) enhance its credibility with purchasers and (2) make more specialty providers available to referring generalists. If it elects not to have its providers responsible for specialty treatment it will need to specify that in both the provider contract and the subscriber contract. The following paragraphs show a good method of handling the situation in a contract. By pointing out that providers should refer patients to the specialty providers in the system so that patients receive as many benefits as possible, it increases DMI Plan's overall appeal to prospective patients.

Specialty Referral. DMI Plans shall supply the Dentist with a list of specialists who are under contract to DMI Plans. All referrals must be made to specialists who are under contract with DMI Plans. If a specialist is needed and DMI Plans does not have a specialist under contract in the specialty required, then the Dentist may refer the Member to the specialist of the Dentist's choice; however, the Dentist must notify the Member that the services of such specialist will not be covered under the contract and the Member will be responsible for the fee charged by that specialist. Should the Dentist fail to notify the Member that the fees will not be covered, the Dentist will be responsible for any difference in the amount of fees charged by the specialist and any co-payment charge that would normally have been paid by the Member under the DMI Plans contract.

Should the Dentist refer a Member to a specialist of the Dentist's choice after having been duly notified in writing by DMI Plans that such a specialist is under contract to provide services under the DMI Plans contract, then the Dentist will be responsible for any difference in the amount of fees charged by the specialist and any co-payment charge that would have normally been paid by the Member under the DMI Plan contract.

Maintaining Credibility

Another good clause to include in the contract is one which further protects the interests of DMI Plans and helps to increase its overall credibility by providing that the office of the dentist is covered in the event he takes an extended vacation. If patients want to visit the office and it is never available to them, the dentist's credibility will once again be tarnished. A sample clause might read as follows:

> Whenever the Dentist is to be absent or away from the office for an extended period of time, the Dentist shall provide a substitute dentist who shall be responsible for the delivery of services under the DMI Plans agreement. In the event the Dentist fails to make necessary arrangements as described above, DMI Plans has the right to obtain services in any manner appropriate for the eligible subscriber and the Dentist shall be responsible for the costs incurred from that action.

Administrative Functions

One of the administrative functions DMI Plans will have to perform is to determine which individual members of the groups it contracts with are eligible for services during the contract period. An employer who may be contributing to the program through matching payroll deductions may not want to begin paying for an individual employee until that employee has proven that he will become a valuable member of his team. One can easily see how the thread of eligibility will have to run from the subscriber contract through the provider contract to establish viability of the entire system. The HMO laws will have some bearing on this issue, as will the federal COBRA law. A method will have to be created to determine who among the members are eligible and then a reporting system will have to be devised to let the dentist know who should receive treatment and who should not. It might be wise to predetermine what will happen if a member is given treatment who is not eligible.

Letting the dentist know who is eligible is most frequently done by the means of an identification card that is presented to the dentist by the patient at the time of treatment. This card is updated as the contracts are updated. In addition, it will be helpful to have a monthly list that can be mailed to the dentist to advise him of changes in eligibility. If questions still arise, provision should be made so that the dentist can call on the phone and get an instantaneous advisory as to the eligibility of an individual.

> **Eligibility.** DMI Plans, in conjunction with any groups or organizations with whom it has contracted, shall make all determinations of eligibility for benefits of any person under this contract, and shall notify the Dentist in advance as to whether or not an individual is entitled to any services pursuant to this contract.

> DMI Plans shall not be liable to the Dentist for any services provided to persons not certified as eligible as herein provided.
>
> DMI Plans shall provide the Dentist with an eligibility list updated monthly from which it can be determined who is eligible for services. If a patient presents for treatment and is not on the list, but claims to be eligible, the Dentist may contact DMI by telephone to ascertain whether said Member is eligible before refusing to provide services under this agreement.

Paying The Providers

The next major issue that we will have to address on our provider contract is the method for paying the dentist. This is capitation. DMI Plans receives a fixed fee every month for each member who signs up for the program. It must then distribute a portion of that fee to the providers in the system. If you or your chain of offices are the only ones involved, the problem is simple. Remove the administration costs, take some for yourself, and give the rest to the dental office. Rarely will it be that simple.

We will discuss the issue of capitation rates in greater detail later. For now assume that DMIPlans has established a fee that will make it viable for a practitioner to join the plan without losing money. That fee is paid on the basis of how many people sign up for a particular dentist. This points directly to the issue of signing up in the subscriber contract. This is one of the hardships of any capitation plan. Can members who sign up for one dental office switch to another midway through the contract? That can cause a variety of problems. Do you establish the provider network in advance by telling the providers that they may get some patients or they may not? Or do you wait to set up the network when you are certain you have enough patients in a given area to provide the volume which will make it practical for a provider to operate under the system?

Regardless, the capitation rate is multiplied by the number of people who sign up for a given office and is paid to that dentist at the beginning or the end of each month depending on whether you float or not. On the contract it might be wise to add this as an "exhibit" so that you can change it or add additional rates depending on what contracts you can negotiate in the future. Wording for this part of the contract might go like this:

> **Basis of Payment to the Dentist.** DMI Plans shall pay to the Dentist the monthly capitation rate described on Exhibit "A" multiplied by the number of eligible participants who select the Dentist as a provider

during the sign-up period of the contract. Such payment shall be made on the thirtieth of each month in which the group or organization makes such capitation payment to DMI Plans as agreed to in the subscriber contract for that organization or group.

In the event that the group does not pay within thirty (30) days after the premium due date, the Dentist may, at will, notify the subscribers that no further services will be performed during the period of premium of delinquency, or that any services performed during the period of delinquency shall be charged at the Dentist's usual, customary, and reasonable fee.

If the group does not bring its premium payments up to date, then DMI Plans will terminate its contract with the group and the Dentist shall have the right to charge all Members who received treatment after the due date of the premium his usual, customary, and reasonable fees.

In no event shall DMI Plans be obligated to pay the Dentist out of its own funds in the event the group does not pay in accordance with its contract.

DMI Plans shall be obligated to notify the Dentist in writing within three (3) days in the event that a group does not pay its premiums on time. In the event DMI Plans fails to give proper notice of delinquent payments then it shall be responsible to pay the Dentist his capitation fee from its own funds.

Fees Due Directly from Member. In the event the Dentist delivers services which are not covered benefits under the contract between the group and DMI Plans, or services which have a co-payment as defined in Exhibit "B," then the Dentist should look to the Member for the applicable fees. In no event shall DMI Plans be responsible to assist the Dentist in collecting said fees.

DMI Plans may, from time to time, raise the applicable co-pays, and will notify the Dentist accordingly.

Exclusions

DMI Plans will want to exclude some things from its provider contract. Some dental treatments do not lend themselves well to prepaid plans. It is impossible under a capitation plan to accurately assess the relative values of some treatments in relation to others, and therefore impossible to justify a reasonable capitation rate and a corresponding co-pay. In addition, a dentist cannot be held responsible for each and every condition that patients may present. Some may even be self- inflicted. Patients may want a treatment simply because they have read about it in a consumer magazine and feel as though it is correct for them. These types of decisions are best made by the dentist and not the patient. That is especially true if the treatment does not have predictable results and cannot be delivered efficiently. Treatment of the TMJ is an example of a treatment where results are unpredictable, yet patients may feel it would benefit them and that they are entitled to the treatment under their plan.

It is important that we insert these types of clauses into the member contract, and then weave them through our provider contract and any other documents where their inclusion would clarify our intent. The list of possible exclusions and limitations in this regard is indefinite. The following are examples of some of the things others have excluded from their plans:

Excusions and Limitations. The Dentist shall not be responsible for:

1. Any dental service not specifically described in the Schedule of Benefits.
2. Any new service or procedure after the last day of the month during which any Member ceased to be eligible for coverage under the group's plan with DMI Plans. Procedures in progress shall be completed. These procedures will include dental treatment where an impression has been taken and/or procedures on any tooth upon which treatment has been started.
3. Visits to or services performed by a specialist, dentist, or professional not authorized by DMI Plans.
4. Any dental services which are necessitated as a result of war or any act of war whether such war be declared or undeclared, any riot, insurrection, or civil disturbance.
5. Any dental services arising out of any sickness or injury arising out of or sustained in the course of any occupation or employment for remuneration or profit, where Member may be eligible for workman's compensation benefits, or any reimbursement through any public program, state or federal, or any program of medical or

dental benefits sponsored and paid for by the federal government or any agency thereof.

6. Any dental services which, in the judgment of the Dentist are not necessary and reasonable for the prevention, correction, or im- provement of a condition.
7. Any dental service which is necessitated as a result of a self-inflicted condition.
8. Any dental services necessitated as a result of a condition sustained in the commission of a felony.
9. Oral surgery requiring the setting of fractures or dislocations.
10. Treatment of cysts or neoplasms.
11. Dispensing of drugs for treatment of oral disease not normally supplied in a dental office.
12. Prescription drugs.
13. Congenital defects.
14. Conditions affecting the temporomandibular joint, including dysfunction and/or malfunction.
15. Any costs or expenses incurred in the event the Member is hospitalized for any dental procedure.
16. Services of an anesthetist or anethesiologist.
17. Any dental charges incurred for the treatment of obesity.
18. Gold or gold foil restorations.
19. Appliances or restoration necessary to increase vertical dimension or to restore an occlusion.
20. Programs or treatments which were in progress prior to the date any person became a Member under this plan.
21. Dental services provided at home or any nursing or rest home.
22. Dental services rendered beyond the scope of a dental license.
23. Services in connection with completion of any insurance-type form or reports to insurance companies, attorneys, other doctors, or anyone else.

24. Replacement costs of dental appliances or products which are lost or stolen.

25. Charges by the Dentist for broken appointments.

26. Special requests by Members for customized techniques differing from standard procedures will be provided at additional fees determined by the Dentist. Patients must bear the difference between the plan fees and the special fees.

27. Treatment of patients who in the Dentist's judgment are un- manageable children or emotionally disturbed adults.

Pick and choose among these exclusions. Some may not be reasonable for your particular plan. You may be able to think of others that are appropriate in your situation. The important thing to remember is that you must weave them through all of your documents and contracts so that parties on both sides of the contract understand exactly what you are offering and what you are not. Take care not to exclude too much though. Otherwise you may end up with a noncompetitive plan which no one will want.

One final word about exclusions. If you are offering a basic service plan which does not contain any provision for specialty referrals, it might be wise to include one final paragraph in your exclusion clauses. It will give the generalists in the system the opportunity to back out of anything that is not within their capabilities. When you think about it, it is not a bad clause to put in any contract. After all, exclusions and limitations are for the protection of the dentists and the administrating company and not necessarily the patients.

> This plan specifically excludes any treatments that are of such complexity that they cannot be performed by the Dentist who is under contract with DMI Plans.

This very important escape clause should be added to every document you print during the operation of your plan if it is a basic one. In spite of it and these other limitations, this is an area where you will have a variety of problems with patients. No matter what you tell them in written form (or verbally for that matter), they will not remember it. At least they will forget it long enough to present some sort of argument in your office. It is the same for any type of dental plan including the indemnifiers. Patients think they have dental insurance. It will pay for everything! How many times have patients told you that their plan pays 100% of everything. As you know, few plans actually do. There are usually limitations, deductibles, co-pays, or something else the patient fails to ealize. It is just a fact of doing business. Accept it and be sure to put these things into all of your contracts so that they are understood by all.

Disclaimer

Since we are on the subject, you might want to add another sort of generalized disclaimer to all of your contracts that is for the protection of DMI Plans and clarifies its position in all of this. It reads as follows:

> **Designation of Services.** DMI Plans shall not (and does not agree nor shall it be required to) perform any dental services or do anything herein (notwithstanding any provisions hereof) that would, under applicable laws and regulations, constitute the practice of dentistry. Any provision of this contract to the contrary notwithstanding, the sole responsibility and obligation of DMI Plans shall be to engage in the design and administration of the Prepaid Dental Program and to use its best efforts to obtain the services of qualified, licensed professionals and their staffs to provide and perform the applicable available dental services to eligible participants. It is expressly agreed that under no circumstances shall DMI Plans ensure that the services of such licensed professionals and their staffs will be available at any time or that the "Available Dental Services" as defined herein will be performed at any time. Further, under no circumstances will DMI Plans be required to indemnify or hold harmless the group or any participant from any cost or expense incurred in procuring any "Available Dental Services" as defined herein. All participants shall be entitled to the scheduled services, but only to the extent that DMI Plans shall have succeeded in obtaining the services of qualified professionals and their staffs to provide the same. The professional services will be provided and available only by the prepaid Dentist designated by DMI Plans.

This is sort of a catchall type of clause, but very valuable. It is mandatory that it be included in any member contract, but it probably wouldn't hurt to include it into a provider contract as well. It is a good idea to try to address as many possible problems that can occur before they do.

Additional Points

In addition to the items we have covered so far in our provider contract, DMI Plans should include a few generic clauses that can be found in most contracts of this type, and are for the most part self-explanatory. It cannot be repeated often enough: if you put it into one document, be sure to include it in all of your others. Some examples are:

Missed Appointments. Any Member who fails to keep an appointment may be charged by the Dentist unless the appointment is cancelled at least 24 hours in advance. The missed appointment charge is not a scheduled benefit under this plan and will be paid directly to the Dentist by the Member. Said charge will not exceed $ _____

Member Notice After Termination of Contract. In the event this contract is terminated by either party, the Dentist agrees that he will notify each Member of a group with whom DMI Plans has an agreement, who presents for treatment, that this contract is no longer in effect. If notice is not given to the Member, then the Dentist will treat that Member and accept payment for his services at charges no more than set forth in the Schedule of Benefits.

Some contracts have an interesting twist to this last paragraph. Some companies have sought to maintain their patients once they have contracted with them and in order to eliminate any chance of competition from the dentist who was formerly a provider in their system, they have specified here that the dentist will not treat any of the former capitation patients. That twist might read like this:

In the event this contract is terminated, the Dentist shall not deliver services to any DMI Plans Member after the effective date of termination. If the Dentist delivers treatment, he agrees to assume responsibility for all costs of delivering said services. Members will be responsible for any co-payments as if this agreement were still in effect. In every respect the Dentist will treat DMI Plans Members as if he were still obligated under this agreement.

The Dentist agrees to forward all x-rays and patient records to a new assigned dentist at either the patient's request or the request of DMI Plans or the new dentist, within thirty (30) days after termination of this agreement.

Work in Progress. In the event of termination of this contract, or termination of the contract between DMI Plans and the group, or loss of eligibility of the Member, the Dentist shall be responsible for completing work started prior to the termination of said contract or contracts, as follows:

1. If an impression has been taken, the Dentist shall complete a denture or partial.
2. Work on each individual tooth which may have been started shall be completed.

Effects of Legislation

It is difficult to say what will happen in the future whenever one deals with ideas and concepts that in some way may be controlled by government employees or elected officials. The new tax laws are a prime example. Suddenly one day, all of the rules under which we operate may change. This is especially true when one deals with prepaid health care. It is an extremely volatile game. The insurance commissions in all of the states have had a great deal of difficulty dealing with these types of plans. Some do not even understand them yet, and still they are certain they want to regulate them. Put this clause into your provider contract:

Effects of Legislation. In the event that legislation or regulations are passed or imposed by any duly constituted authority which affect the terms and conditions of this agreement, or the prepaid dental plas offered by DMI Plans, then the parties to this agreement shall promptly attempt to comply with the provisions of such legislation by amending and revising this agreement. In the event compliance with such legislation or regulations is attempted, but the parties to this agreement are unable to accomplish such compliance within a reasonable time, then this agreement shall terminate without further obligation of either of the parties to the other, except for the payment of any money which may then be due and owing.

Practice of Dentistry

Since we are on the subject of laws and regulations, we should put in a clause that further helps to protect DMI Plans in the event the dentist decides to do something controversial.

Practice of Dentistry. The Dentist, his agents and employees, shall at all times comply with the act within the provisions of the state laws relating to the practice of dentistry, licensing, regulation and the practice, licensing, and regulation of hygienists. In the event such laws are amended, added to or revised in the future, the Dentist shall comply and act within such additions, amendments, and revisions.

You might want to take this a bit further at this point and provide some additional protection for your contracted clients, and help to increase your overall credibility with the potential groups with whom you intend to contract.

Standard of Care. The Dentist shall in no way differentiate in the quality of treatment, days of treatment, or time of day of treatment, between DMI Plans Members and his own private patients.

Inclusion of the Dentist on the panel of providers is not necessarily a recommendation of said Dentist by DMI Plans.

A situation may arise in which an individual provider included in your program may have difficulty with a particular patient. Some people simply cannot get along with one another. This may be particularly true in the dentist-patient relationship. Some provider contracts mandate that the dentist treat the patients sent to him by the capitation company no matter what the circumstances. They at least dictate that the dentist pay for the care of the individuals if he cannot treat them. This is unpopular with dentists and can be a matter of contention in the future.

It might be a better idea to include an escape clause for the dentist in the event that he cannot treat a particular individual, and then use our termination clause later if the dentist invokes the clause too often.

Dentists are by nature a self-directed group. They do not enjoy any outside parties interfering with the way they operate their offices, and especially with the way they treat patients. DMI Plans does not really want to get involved in these affairs anyway, so this would be a good place to add some words that ease the dentist's mind and specify who makes decisions of this type.

Dental Relationships. The relationship between the Member and the Dentist shall be subject to the rules, limitations, and privileges incident to the doctor-patient relationship. The Dentist shall be solely responsible to the Member for the advice and treatment of said Member, without interference from DMI Plans or any of its agents.

The Dentist has the right to refuse treatment to any patient who violates the dentist-patient relationship. The Dentist must notify DMI Plans immediately of its intention to invoke provisions of this section. In the event the Dentist refuses to treat a particular Member, rights to future capitation payments for that patient shall be considered waived.

The operation and maintenance of the dental office, facilities and equipment and the rendering of all dental services shall be solely and exclusively under the supervision of the Dentist. DMI Plans shall have no right or authority over the selection or supervision of staff, operation of the dental office, or delivery of dental services. DMI Plans shall have no rights to manage or control the dental office or the delivery of services.

DMI Plans shall not be liable for an act or omission of the Dentist or any of its agents or other persons performing a service at the request of the Dentist.

While DMI Plans does not really want to get involved in the operation of the dental office and does not want to control the activities of the dentist totally, it is still necessary that it monitors and looks out for the interests of its clients. Indeed, one of the functions DMI Plans will provide is to collect utilization information so that fees and capitation rates can be monitored. This is usually accomplished with some type of treatment encounter form. DMI Plans will want to know other types of information such as the frequency of specialty referrals and the amounts of co-payments paid directly to the dentist. It will have to draft forms for this purpose and teach the dentist how to use them. Usually the capitation company will send a representative to the dentist's office who will spend some time explaining procedures to the dentist and the staff. One company which operated in the Midwest for a short period even went so far as to establish a school which was to be attended by the individual practitioners who signed up as providers.

Peer Review

In addition to this type of monitoring, DMI Plans may want to establish a peer review panel which will monitor the appropriateness and quality of the treatment rendered by the dentist. Indeed, state insurance commissions may insist that some form of quality control program is instituted. It seems strange, though, that the administrators of the plans are the ones who choose the members of the review boards. Nonetheless, it is important to specify this in the provider contract.

> **Dental Review Panel.** DMI Plans shall designate and approve all forms, including specialty referral forms, treatment encounter forms, quarterly report forms, and the methods of collection of statistical information. The Dentist agrees to use said forms and follow policies developed by DMI Plans for use of such forms. The Dentist agrees that he has been advised of all procedures and policies and has received a copy of necessary patient encounter forms.
>
> DMI Plans may appoint a Dental Review Panel, made up of licensed dentists who shall advise and assist DMI Plans in the supervision of standards of dental care, matters which relate to the dental-patient relationship, methods and manners of operation, and costs and dental necessity of dental services provided by Dentist contracting with DMI Plans. The decision of the Dental Review Panel shall be final and binding on both parties hereto.

Exclusivity

Another point of contention that should be addressed in your provider contract relates to exclusivity. Some capitation companies seek to ensure that their plan is the only one the dentist handles. Presumably, this limits the dentist's activities in the prepaid market to only their patients, thereby ensuring that their clients will receive more attention. It also may have value in combating competition from other companies which may want to move into their area of operation. It does not sit particularly well with dentists. They resent being told they cannot do something as much as being told they have to do something. Wording for this type of restriction might read like this:

> **Exclusivity.** The Dentist agrees that the Dentist will not, without the written consent of DMI Plans, enter into a contract to provide dental service for any other capitation program or preferred provider organization.

Other capitation companies have held the opinion that in order to ensure the best for their clients, dentists in the system should be as financially viable as possible. If participation in other plans adds to that economic stability, so much the better. The decision about financial matters for his own practice is left up to the dentist. The potential problem is that the dentist will contract with too many groups in an effort to increase his volume and thereby his profits, to the point where he will be spread too thin and not be able to deliver services adequately. This tendency to over-subscribe capitation plans has resulted in failures. In many offices, the problem can be eliminated by the addition of an associate.

You can see how this can be traced back to the office questionnaire. If the office you have chosen to be a provider has no capacity for the addition of an associate, you may want your contract to be exclusive.

For the most part, financial viability is a stronger motivator. Most dentists who consider capitation also will consider an associate and understand the difficulties with over-subscribing, rendering the question moot. You can tell the dentist that it is okay for him to enter into other contracts like this:

> **Nonexclusivity.** This contract is mutually nonexclusive. DMI Plans, participating groups or organizations, or individual members of such groups are entitled to enter into similar contracts with other dentists. The Dentist is also free to enter into other contracts with other capitation companies, other groups, and any others not represented by DMI Plans, and to maintain his private practice as well.

Miscellaneous Clauses

Here are a few additional clauses that should be incorporated into your capitation provider contracts. Most of them are self-explanatory:

> **Advertising.** In the event the Dentist advertises in any manner whatsoever, the Dentist shall not use the DMI Plans name without first and on each occasion obtaining DMI Plans' written consent.

> **Confidential Information.** The Dentist acknowledges that DMI Plans has invested substantial time, expertise, and expense in creating prepaid dental plan documentation. The Dentist agrees that this documentation is the property of DMI Plans and will be kept confidential and used by the Dentist only for the purposes for which it is devised.

> **Modification and Assignability.** This agreement contains the entire and complete understanding between the parties. This agreement shall not be assignable by the parties hereto or performed by anyone except the parties, without the written consent of the other.

Or, if you want to prevent the dentist from assigning the contract to someone else, perhaps in the event of the sale of his practice, and still retain your rights to sell your capitation business and its contracts to another interested party, you might use assignability wording like this:

> Because of the nature of the services to be performed, this agreement shall not be assignable by the Dentist, nor shall the benefits thereof be passed on to and naturalized by the Dentist's heirs and/or successors in interest. DMI Plans shall be entitled to assign this agreement to its heirs, representatives, successors and/or assigns without limitation.

A clause like this one will help to protect your clients and further ensure your credibility.

> **Claims Against Members.** Under no circumstances will the Dentist, or his agents, or representatives, whether employed directly or indirectly, make any charges or claims against a Member for any services rendered, which by this contract will be compensated by the manner described herein, except for any charge which is to be made directly to the Dentist under the terms of this contract.

To avoid further costs involved with legal affairs, it might be a good idea to handle any disputes which may arise by means of arbitration as opposed to civil actions.

> **Disputes.** In the event any dispute arises between the parties of this agreement, it is agreed that said dispute shall be settled by arbitration in accordance with the rules and regulations, then in effect, of the American Arbitration Association. Any judgment or award rendered by the arbitrator may be duly entered into any court, having jurisdiction thereof. The prevailing party shall be entitled to costs and reasonable attorney's fees.

Two more odds and ends should be included as follows:

Dental Records. All dental records for Members of groups contracting with DMI Plans shall be retained by the Dentist for a period of at least five (5) years after the date of said Member's last visit to the office. DMI Plans and/or its agents or representatives shall be entitled to inspect said records upon reasonable written request.

Notices. Whenever it becomes necessary for either party to serve notice on the other respecting the terms of this contract, such notice shall be served by certified mail, return receipt requested, addressed as indicated below.

Closing

All that is left is the signatures and attachments, and we will have the basis of a provider contract for a dental capitation plan.

IN WITNESS WHEREOF, the parties to this contract have affixed their signatures in duplicate on this _____ day of _________ , 19 __________

Dentist	**DMI Plans**
by: ________________________	**by:** ________________________

Address ______________________

City/State ____________________

ZIP Code _____________________

Phone _______________________

State License No. ______________

Attachments: capitation rate, description of various plans, co-pay rates.

Do not copy the individual segments of this chapter and expect to use them as a contract for capitation in your state. It is mandatory that you seek the services of a licensed attorney to determine specifically what is required in your state, and to put the various elements into the correct perspective for your particular contract. Use them instead as guides, to formulate your own ideas about capitation contracts before you contact your lawyer. You may want to delete some of these clauses and add others.

It is our purpose here to dissect the various aspects of a provider contract and thereby educate the reader. No intention is made here to provide an actual contract.

Patient Encounter Forms

One other item will be necessary as part of the printed armamentarium for administration of your capitation plan. Its necessity is something of an irony. One selling point of pre-paid plans to both the potential subscribers as well as the providers is the lack of paperwork. "There are no complicated insurance forms to deal with when you sign up for DMI Plans," they say. But in reality there are—at least to the provider. The HMO law, and, no doubt, the insurance commission regulations in your state will require DMI Plans to keep some sort of record with regards to individual patient visits to the dental office. Indeed, DMI Plans itself will benefit by some sort of monitoring of utilization so that it can have a better idea of what kinds of groups it intends to contract with and how much to charge them for capitation rates. Such records will also enable DMI Plans to provide information to prospective providers as to what kind of increases in patient visits their participation in your plans will make in their offices. The irony is that the dentist must still fill out a form which in most respects is similar to any insurance form, and requires almost as much time to fill out. It will have to be a responsibility of one or more auxiliaries in the dental office and thereby will contribute to the overall expense of the program. Additionally, DMI Plans will have to arrange for compliance with this requirement each month, much in the same manner that it informs the dentist about eligibility of participants. That will increase its costs as well. But no matter, someone's got to do it!

The standard patient encounter form can be modeled after a typical spreadsheet formula. At the top, there should be some spaces to fill-in particular information about a given participant, the group to which he belongs, his identification number, the provider's name and the date. It will helpful to gather information about each specific tooth that is treated at a particular visit, so below the identification information, the procedures covered by your plan should be listed. On the left, in column form, the teeth should be listed. Some companies have merely listed types of services like "Filling" or "Root canal." Others are more specific and list all of the various procedures listed in any standard ADA fee-service schedule. The more specific information you are able to gather, the more uses you will be able to make of it later. One such use will be to convince groups of the viability of your plan when it comes time to sign them to another contract, or when attempting to solicit new business from other groups. If you can point out to a particular group that in the preceding year the members of their group received X-number of fillings which when multiplied by standard fees would have cost so many dollars, but since they were members of DMI Plans, they paid only this much, and so on, it will act as a strong sales aid.

This gridded spreadsheet format is easy to use. An auxiliary using a ruler can simply check a box or two and provide much information about a particular patient visit.

A patient encounter form might look like this:

COMMENTS:

NAME: __________

Group #: __________

Employer: __________

Primary Subscriber: __________

Date: __________

Tooth	Initial Oral Exam	Periodic Oral Exam	Emergency Office Call	X-rays - Any Type	Cleaning	Flouride Treatments	Space Maintainers	Fillings -Silver	Fillings - White	Incisal Edge Filling	Pin Core - Any Material	Post Core Cost/Preformed	Stainless Steel Crown	Inlay and Onlays	Full Crowns - Any Metal	Porcelain To Metal Crown	Pulpotomy	Apical Closure	Root Canal	Apical Curretage	Occlusal Adjustments	Root Planning & Curretage	Gingivectomy	Specialized Perio	Simple Extraction	Additional Tooth	Surgical Extraction	Soft Tissue Impaction	Partial Bony Impaction	Complete Bony Impaction	Ostioplasty	Complete Dentures	Partials	Relines
N/A																																		
1																																		
2																																		
3																																		
4																																		
5																																		
6																																		
7																																		
8																																		
9																																		
10																																		
11																																		
12																																		
13/A																																		
14/B																																		
15/C																																		
16/D																																		
17/E																																		
18/F																																		
19/G																																		
20/H																																		
21/I																																		
22/J																																		
23/K																																		
24/L																																		
25/M																																		
26/N																																		
27/O																																		
28/P																																		
29/Q																																		
30/R																																		
31/S																																		
32/T																																		

Chapter 7 Subscriber Relations

We are now ready to begin thinking about dealing with the actual people who will become patients under our plan. We need to think about how to define and solicit them. We will need to contract with them somehow, and we must manage their accounts once they are members. And, no matter who they turn out to be and what type of arrangement we will ultimately make with them, one of the first things they will want to know is what this plan is going to cost them. Incidentally, this is one of the first things the insurance commission will want to know as well. From a practical standpoint, fees and contracting with the subscribers are two of the most important considerations in the entire concept of prepaid dentistry.

Establishing Fees

Dental capitation requires the establishment of two basic fees (1) the monthly premium rate or capitation rate paid by subscribers or their employers or unions and (2) the fees the patients will actually have to pay when they receive treatment, or the co-pay fees. The HMO Act of 1973 addresses this topic somewhat and establishes a couple of parameters for rate development. The law says that each member is to be provided services for a payment which shall be:

1. Paid on a periodic basis without regard to the date on which the services is actually rendered
2. Fixed without regards to frequency, or extent of service
3. Determined by the community rating system

The act goes on to justify the establishment of co-pays which come directly out of the pocket of the patient by saying that the capitation rates outlined above may be supplemented by additional nominal payments for specific services. The act qualifies that by giving power to the insurance commissioners to determine that a specific co-pay may not be applicable if that fee would act as a deterrent to actual delivery of a service by being out of affordable range for patients.

The Community Rating System

The first two guidelines for rate determination are self- explanatory. The third, regarding the community rating system, deserves closer scrutiny. It is to be distinguished from its antithesis: the experience rating system. Under the community rating system, all subscribers under the plan are to be charged the same fee. Nominal differences are allowed between individuals, small groups, and larger groups depending upon marketing considerations, but basically the capitation rate must be equal in each instance that the plan is offered within a specific community. The experience rating system allows different fees to be charged based upon actuarial statistics which determine the frequency with which a certain group will require or use a specific service. Insurance companies use this method for determining their rates. It gives them a specific marketing advantage over the HMOs in that they can charge lower rates to those groups expected to have a low claim rate based on prevailing health. Under the experience rating system, less healthy groups will pay higher rates than healthy groups. Under the community rating system, healthy groups bear the cost of supporting unhealthy groups. Redistribution of wealth seems to be the ubiquitous mandate of legislatures. Nonetheless, when designing capitation plans you must use the community rating system.

Dental Capitation Rate Formulas

Determining the actual capitation rate charged to groups for basic dental services is not easy. Gray areas within the formula make it speculative in many cases. It depends too on the viewpoint of the person establishing the rate. Some investigators have said that the rate per person should equal the anticipated hours a dentist must devote to a capitation patient times the cost of those hours. Sounds simple, doesn't it? The number of hours times the hourly rate equals the capitation rate. In reality, many factors cloud the simplicity of the equation.

Most notably, the hourly cost is not fixed. Consider the hourly cost of the doctor's chair time and the hourly cost of the hygienist's chair time. Consider too, diferences in the efficiency from one doctor to another and differences in efficiency within an office at different times. Some patients require more time than others and some may require procedures others do not. Setting rates based on cost of operation has another drawback in that it assumes only a "break-even" point. If the rate is based on the hourly or monthly cost of providing services, nothing is left over for profit. If the providers must rely on only those excess revenues received from participants who do not show for treatment, it will not take long for him to lose respect for the system and begin to incorporate some of the policies that have met with the greatest criticism of capitation in general. To add a profit figure to the cost equation may be difficult since valuing the worth of a particular doctor's services may be a perplexing undertaking.

In addition, some have argued that if you treat a capitation patient, you will not be able to treat a fee-for-service patient during that time slot. Therefore, a factor must be added to the equation that accounts for that less-than-ideal chair time. If that is a consideration for you, perhaps you should re-evaluate whether participation in capitation plans is a wise decision for you in the first place. Remember, we said that if you have no free chair time and suspect that trend will continue for a long time, why accept any capitation patients? For you, adding capitation will mean adding staff, equipment, and overall hours of operation to handle the additional load. Start slow, work a few capitation patients into your schedule only if you have the time. Gearing up to incorporate a program you do not need may be a costly venture.

Analyzing rate structures based on cost faces another serious obstacle. Costs of treating capitation patients and the revenue received from them may not necessarily parallel one another. Typically, utilization of the program will be high at first, while revenues will lag behind. At the beginning of a plan, providers will be forced to absorb most of the costs of operation. Hopefully as the contract enters the later stages of its duration, the patients will have been treated and the provider will make up his loss by not having to provide treatment while continuing to receive the capitation rate. It doesn't always work out that way. Experience dictates that towards the end of a contract period a provider can once again expect a surge of patients who have waited until the last minute to seek treatment. This can be a particularly frustrating experience for the provider because these patients are often very demanding about the delivery of that service before the end of the contract period. They do not necessarily view dentistry as an ongoing process but tend to assume that it is a one-time adventure, and have no intention of re-signing in the subsequent year. This dilemma of cost/revenue lag points towards longer contract periods for subscribers which will give the providers an opportunity to enjoy the good along with the bad. We will discuss that again when we discuss subscriber contracts.

A Place to Start

Regardless of where you find yourself in this madness, you must nevertheless come up with a rate. A good way to start is to calculate a rate based on past performance. This method is more predictable and takes into consideration what you would have made treating other patients and your costs as well. You will need to know the total gross production of an office in a year and the numbers of family units seen during that time. A family unit could be an individual or an actual family. Since capitation plan enrollees are made up of individuals and family groups, what is important is to try to correlate the numbers to potential subscribers of your plan. From the total gross production, you can subtract the laboratory expenses since most capitation plans include sufficient co-pays to cover laboratory bills, and those costs are born by recipients directly. Once you have this modified production figure, you must divide it by the total number of family units (subscribers). This will give a figure that describes what the average charge to patients was during a year. Divide this by 12 and you will have a figure that represents a capitation rate that allows economic viability for the provider in your example. But just in case, do a cost evaluation as a counter check. Compute the total expenses of the office (less lab bills and doctor salaries). Divide that by the number of family units, and again by 12, and you will have an idea of the cost incurred in treating those patients in a year. It should be less than capitation rate, and the ratio between the two could predict the relative profit a provider could expect in a similar circumstance. If utilization is less than 100%, which it usually is, a provider could expect a greater profit. If he is increasingly cost conscious, profits could rise even farther.

If you are designing a rate to be used by a group of offices, in an IPA, for example, or just a group wishing to start a capitation plan for itself, you will have to take an average of these numbers from all of the offices in the system to use in your calculations. If you are an administrator charged with developing this rate, you will be at a disadvantage unless you can obtain these numbers from some cooperative source. Perhaps you can obtain them from the dental management magazines available at any library or subscribe to the National Dental Fee Survey Company, P.O. Box 1715, Des Plaines, Illinois 60017. They can provide lists of current fees used by dentists anywhere in the country which can be broken down into regions and even ZIP codes.

To this base rate that must be paid to the providing offices, you must add your administrative costs. These are the marketing and operational costs plus the profit your administration companywill want. Here again calculation of these costs will take some consideration. Project everything you can possibly imagine for the groups you intend to solicit and then add some for incidentals and errors. Here is where the self-administered plan should have superiority over the third party-administered plan. If you can cut out the middleman, you should be able to offer a rate that is considerably lower and therefore much more competitive.

One last complication satisfied by this method of rate formulation is that at first you will not know how many people will sign up fr a particular office. If you set your rate based on the cost of treating a fixed number of patients without knowing how many people that will actually mean, it could result in a gross calculation error in either direction. If you have a group of 100 families and four doctors to treat them, random distribution would predict that each practitioner would receive 25 families in his practice. In reality, one man may get fifty and the other three could divide the remainder. Predicting the rate based on past in-house experience will mean that each practitioner could still profit regardless of the actual numbers of subscribers.

You may want to establish a flexible rate schedule instead of a fixed one. Without question, higher utilization rates are to be expected with smaller groups. Therefore you may want to reduce the rate for those larger groups interested in your plan. The trick will be justifying the variable rate within the restriction of the community rating system. With computerization actual administration costs may not be that much different if the size of the group rises, so you can usually afford to do it assuming the difference will be offset by lower utilization rates. If you are an administrative company only, there is no question you can do it since utilization expense will be borne by the providers anyway.

Finally, just before you make your presentation of the rate to the groups you are intending to sign up, take a look around. See what your competitors are charging. Capitation rates are like any other commodity. They are based ultimately on what the traffic will bear.

Co-pay Fees

The HMO Act delineates the general purpose of capitation to be the provision of basic and supplemental health services for a fixed periodic rate. That rate can be complemented only nominally by additional payments from patients for some specific services. In dentistry, that has come to mean that most preventive and restorative procedures do not have a co-payment assigned to them. Because the act gives the power to decide if a particular fee should be allowed or not to the commissioners this is an area of possible negotiation when you are applying for licensure. Obviously, the higher the co-pays for services, the more attractive the plan will be to providers. Traditionally with prepaid plans, as co-pays rise, capitation rates decline and vice versa.

An underlying principle to establishing co-pays is that they should be low on those procedures which are the least expensive to deliver, and more on those services which are costly to deliver. Clearly, those procedures involving laboratory bills should contain co-pays that are at least as high as those bills. It is not unreasonable to add co-pay amounts for those services which are associated with increased labor on the part of a dentist. A root canal, for example, requires extensive chair time on the part of the dentist, and therefore deserves some sort of co-pay. A crown has a laboratory bill associated with it and is labor-intensive as well. Therefore, its corresponding co-pay should reflect both of these charges. Placing a band-and-loop spacer in a child's mouth is not a labor-intensive procedure. One only needs to take a quick alginate impression and on a subsequent visit cement it into place. It does, however, involve a laboratory charge, and needs a co-pay to offset that. Some plans charge only a "laboratory fee" as a co-pay and merely pass the charge on to the patient. Others charge according to a table of allowances based on averaging laboratory fees for a particular procedure.

Co-pays for preventive procedures are historically low for several reasons. First of all, they are the least expensive procedures for the provider to perform. Indeed, many providers have already entered into some sort of advertising campaign which offers discounts on these services in hopes of attracting new patients. It does not cost very much for a doctor to do an exam. Nor is there a great deal of cost involved in X-rays. If you break them down to individual films, you will find they carry one of the greatest markups in all of consumerism. So too with fluoride. On a per application basis, the profit ratio is exceptional. Some labor and chair time is involved when performing a prophy however, and therefore it is not unreasonable to charge a small co-pay for that service. That is especially true if it is a difficult prophy or borders on periodontal treatment like the curettage and scaling procedures.

Another reason co-pays on preventive procedures are low is that from a providers standpoint, one of the goals of the entire capitation concept is to take a group of patients and raise their collective dental health to a level where they do not need treatment. Under that ideal situation, the providers can enter into the best of all possible worlds where they are receiving the capitation fees each month but are not required to deliver any services for them. It is an idealistic view, because it seldom works quite that way, but this is the basic idea. Make the prevention inexpensive, and you might not have to provide services later. Certainly this is one of the legislative precepts for the entire capitation movement. It is without question one of the governing argumens offered by proponents of cost containment.

Low co-pays on prevention has a practical aspect from a marketing standpoint. If you are in the business of selling prepaid plans, it will be much easier if you can convince prospective clients that joining your plan and paying the capitation rate each month will save them money. Let's assume you are speaking to a mother of three children. Assume too that no one in her family has ever needed a root canal or a crown. She knows that she and the kids should go to the dentist every six months to have their teeth cleaned and checked to prevent minor problems from becoming major. The problem for her is that for the four of them to go just once for routine maintenance under a fee-for-service basis could cost in the neighborhood of $250. And if dad decides to go as well, it would be even more. And while she knows she should do it, it may be difficult to fit that bill into the budget. You can bet she will remember what that simple preventive visit will cost, while she may be totally unaware of what it will cost to have a root canal or a crown performed. If your capitation rates are acceptable and can be paid on a monthly basis either directly or through payroll deductions, or better yet, if someone else like an employer or a trust fund is paying for them, she may decide to take your program on just the basis of your prevention co-pays and you will have made a sale!

Co-pays for treatments that require the services of a specialist may have to be somewhat higher. Remember from our discussion of provider contracts that dealing with the specialists may involve particular problems. In order to assure that you will be able to attract some of them to your program, it will be necessary to have high co-pays. Having specialists in your program is important both from the standpoint of logistics and from that all-important credibility battle.

One last reminder about co-pays. As is true with your capitation rates, it will benefit you to take a look at what the competition is offering. You are in a competitive business, and if you are marketing your plan, you will have to offer either a competitive price or a unique service worth more than customary fees.

Targeting Subscriber Contracts

The prepaid concept involves two promises. The patients promise to pay the capitation rate monthly (or periodically) and the doctors promise to deliver the services. Linking those two promises requires a contract. Before you can write the contract, you must understand who is actually making the promises. On the doctor side of the equation, it is actually the capitation company who contracts with patients and not the doctors directly. They are linked to the capitation company through the provider contract. On the patient side, it is not their promise that must be linked, but rather the promise of whoever is going to actually pay the premium. So we have payer versus capitation company, not patient versus doctor.

This payer can take on many forms. In its most simple form it is the employer who agrees to pay the entire capitation rate as an employee benefit. It may however take on a more complicated identity. The capitation rate could be part employer contribution, part employee contribution through payroll deductions, part union contribution, part trust fund contribution, part defined benefit package contribution and so on. Ironically, it is when the payer takes on the form of an individual patient paying his own capitation rate that most problems for capitation companies (and doctors) develop. For the discussion of subscriber contracts to follow, let's assume that we are following our rule of keeping it simple and small by directing our efforts towards a small company with 100 or so employees. Let's further assume that we will be receiving one capitation check from the employer each month, instead of many checks from individuals or other parties. The employer writes one check comprised of both his contribution and the contribution of his employee through payroll deductions. The check is calculated by taking the capitation rate times the numbers of subscribers in the plan.

Subscriber Contracts

Capitation contracts, you will remember, are collections of ideas that can be traced back through the HMO laws, state regulations, provider contracts, marketing materials, and all other aspects of the business.

Opening

Our contract should start out in the usual way by specifying exactly who the parties on both sides of the promises are. The opening might read as follows:

Dental Maintenance International
Contract Agreement

THIS CONTRACT AGREEMENT made and entered into this _______ day of ______________________, 19 ___, by and between DENTAL MAINTENANCE INTERNATIONAL, INC. (hereinafter referred to as "DMI"), and ___________________________________, (hereinafter referred to as the "Master Subscriber").

Notice that it is the employer and not the individual patients with whom we are contracting. For our subscriber contract, the recitals might read something like this:

Recitals

Witnesseth:

WHEREAS, DENTAL MAINTENANCE INTERNATIONAL, INC. has arranged for the services of qualified, licensed professionals and their staffs to participate in a prepaid dental plan, and

WHEREAS, the Master Subscriber desires to enroll as a member and subscribe to the prepaid dental plan offered by DENTAL MAINTENANCE INTERNATIONAL, INC.

NOW, THEREFORE, in consideration of the mutual covenants, conditions and promises contained herein, it is agreed upon between the parties as follows:

1. The Master Subscriber is hereby accepted as a member of the Prepaid Dental Plan offered by DENTAL MAINTENANCE INTERNATIONAL, INC.
2. The Master Subscriber hereby accepts and agrees to the provisions, terms, and conditions set forth in this agreement. It is agreed that

all rights and obligations of each party to the other shall be governed exclusively by the provisions of this agreement.

3. The Master Subscriber hereby agrees to offer this plan to all eligible members of the group and to make periodic payments to DMI on behalf of those members who elect to join the plan as described in this agreement.

4. DMI agrees to arrange for the provision of services for members according to the terms of this agreement.

Definitions

When examining subscriber group contracts, it is possible to find a great variety of terms that could apply to your situation. A few are listed below. Be sure to use this section of the contract to define anything which later could be a point of contention in the event some sort of legal action is necessary. Alternative definitions are given for some of the terms.

Definitions of Certain Terms Used Herein

1. Contract Agreement. The agreement executed by DENTAL MAINTENANCE INTERNATIONAL, INC., hereinafter referred to as "DMI" and the applicable Group Master Subscriber.

2. Contract Month. A calendar month while each respective Contract Agreement is in effect.

3. Contract Year. A period of twelve (12) Contract Months.

4. Master Subscriber. The employer, union, or organization that executes the Contract Agreement in conjunction with DMI.

5. Eligible Member. The employee of an employr group, member of an association, union, or other organization who is deemed eligible for coverage under the plan by the Master Subscriber and is herein described.

6. Enrollee or Member. A person entitled to receive dental services under this Master Contract through the Contract Agreement of the Master Subscriber.

7. Enrollee Services. Professional services available to an enrollee with respect to himself or his eligible dependents.

8. Eligible Dependent. The lawful husband or wife of an enrollee (herein called the spouse) if no judicial decree of separation has been obtained, and such of the unmarried children of the enrollee from birth to the age of nineteen (19), or such of the unmarried children as are between the ages of nineteen (19) to twenty-three (23), and who are classified as full-time students at an accredited educational institution. For purposes of the preceding sentence, the term "educational institution" shall mean only an educational institution which normally maintains a regular faculty and curriculum and normally has a regularly organized body of students in attendance at the place where its educational activities are carried on.

9. Provider. A Dentist or Dental Specialist operating within the scope of his license, and/or other person qualified and authorized to perform dental treatment under the laws of the State.

10. Contracted Dental Service. Any service or treatment delivered by or under the direction of a Dentist which is essential for the necessary dental care of a enrollee, but only if it is listed in the Schedule of Dental Services and performed in accordance with the Dental Maintenance International, Inc. Prepaid Dental Plan.

11. Provider. The Dentists and other providers who have an arrangement with DMI to perform dental services for the Master Subscriber.

12. Capitation Rate. The monthly charges which the Master Subscriber or the Enrollees will be responsible for paying in order to maintain coverage under this contract.

13. Precovered Benefits. Means provider services, the cost of which are included in the Capitation rate.

14. Co-Payment Services. Provider services the cost of which is to be paid directly by the Enrollee.

15. Co-Payment Charges. The amount which an enrollee will be responsible for paying to the Provider performing co-payment services.

Standard Disclaimer and Designation of Services

At this point in our contract it might be wise to designate exactly what it is that DMI will do. It is pretty much the standard disclaimer that we used in our provider contract. Its intent is to insulate DMI from having to actually provide dental services and advises that our function is only that of a negotiator trying to find providers for the plan.

Designation of Services. On behalf of the Master Subscriber, DMI has arranged for the services of qualified, licensed Providers and their staffs to participate in the Prepaid Dental Program herein described. The Master Subscriber shall be entitled to those services described in the Schedule of Benefits, a copy of which is attached hereto and incorporated by this reference.

DMI shall not (and does not agree nor shall it be required to) perform any dental services or do anything herein (notwithstanding any provisions hereof) that would, under applicable laws and regulations, constitute the practice of dentistry. Any provision of this agreement to the contrary notwithstanding, the sole responsibility and obligation of DMI shall be to engage in the design and administration of the Prepaid Dental Program and to use its best efforts to obtain the services of qualified, licensed Providers and their staffs to provide and perform the applicable Contracted Dental Services to eligible enrollees. It is expressly agreed that under no circumstances shall DMI ensure that the services of such licensed providers and their staffs will be available at any time or that the "Contracted Dental Services" as defined herein will be performed at any time. Further, under no circumstances will DMI be required to indemnify or hold harmless the Master Subscriber or any Enrollee from any cost or expense incurred in procuring any Contracted Dental Services as defined herein. All Enrollees shall be entitled to the scheduled services, but only to the extent that DMI shall have succeeded in obtaining the services of qualified providers and their staffs to provide the same. The provider services will be provided and available only by the Provider designated by DMI.

Eligibility

The HMO Act generally outlines to whom you must offer your plan and how they will become eligible. To paraphrase for our purposes here, you must offer it to every member of the group and cannot rule out anyone on the basis of existing health or anything else. It does, however, make some references to the age and status of children dependents not attending accredited colleges. The definitions section of our contract covers this general eligibility criterion. However, an employer may want to add some additional qualifiers for people in his particular group. For example, an employer who is paying all or part of an employee's capitation rate under this plan may be reluctant to pay the fee for an employee who may not remain in his organization for very long. If he takes on a new employee, he may want to wait for a while to see if it is going to be worth it to pay additional premiums should the employee be terminated shortly after hiring. Or, he may not want to pay the capitation rate for temporary or part-time employees. Or, in the case where the group is a member of an association of some kind, the association might want its members to fulfill a waiting period or other eligibility requirement to assure viability as a member.

This part of the contract is negotiable, and so should contain some blanks to be filled in after discussions with the prospective employer.

In our contract it might read something like this:

Eligibility. The eligibility of individual Members shall be determined as follows:

1. Eligible Members shall include:

   a. All full-time employees working a minimum of _____ hours

   or

   b. All employees (or members in the case of an association) in good standing

   or

   c. Other: ____

2. It is hereby agreed that the applicable waiting period for an employee entering the service of the Master Subscriber after the effective date of this agreement shall be the first of the month following _______ months of service.

3. Dependents eligible to become Enrollees are those designated in the definition section of this agreement. No dependent of any Eligible Member shall be eligible to become an Enrollee of the Prepaid Dental Plan unless such Eligible Member shall first have satisfied the waiting period requirement, if applicable.

If when you are customizing your contract with the group you are intending to sign up, you decide that a waiting period is not necessary, simply write the paragraph something like this:

Each eligible member designated by the Master Subscriber as eligible shall be able to elect participation on the effective date of the plan, without a waiting period.

Participation

In addition to describing the parameters of eligibility, it is important to outline how an employee can join the plan. Just because he suddenly becomes eligible does not necessarily mean he has to join. Capitation plans are voluntary, and we want to make sure it is clear the employee has elected to become a member by his own choice. This is usually accomplished by means of an open enrollment period, but you may find it necessary to make available different methods for participation if an employer insists that members becoming eligible after the sign-up period can still enter the plan. We will discuss the logistics of sign-up in greater detail when we discuss marketing in the next chapter. Our contract, however, might address the subject of participation of eligible members and their dependents like this:

Participation. Eligible Members may participate in the plan under the following conditions:

1. Except as otherwise specified, an Eligible Member will become an Enrollee for services on the day he becomes eigible for such services provided:

    a. The Eligible Member completes a written application as specified by DMI, not later than thirty (30) days after he becomes eligible. If the Eligible Member does not sign said written application within the specified period, he must wait until the next open enrollment period to become an Enrollee.

   b. The applicable payment shall have been made by the Master Subscriber with respect to the Eligible Member as of the date such person becomes an Enrollee.

2. Eligible Dependents shall become Enrollees only if:

   a. The requirements of participation 1-a and 1-b above have been satisfied by the Eligible Member.

   b. Said Eligible Dependent has been specifically included on the application form.

   c. Master Subscriber has paid the applicable Capitation Rate for them.

3. Dependents who become eligible after the Eligible Member becomes an Enrollee can only become Enrollees themselves if:

   a. The Enrollee shall have filed a written election with DMI that such Eligible Dependents become Enrollees within thirty (30) days after such Dependents become eligible, on the forms prescribed by DMI.

   b. The Master Subscriber shall have paid the applicable monthly charge in respect to such Dependents.

4. Eligible Dependents who could have become Enrollees on the date the Eligible Member first became an Enrollee, but were not included on the application by the Eligible Member, must wait until the next open enrollment period, as designated by DMI, to enroll. In no event shall dependent services be available if the Eligible Member is not an Enrollee.

5. The initial open enrollment period will begin thirty (30) days prior to the effective date of this agreement. Additional open enrollment periods will be held at the discretion of DMI.

Agreement to Remain In the Plan

When dental capitation plans first became popular, for the most part, they required participants to remain in the plan for a period of one year. It was assumed that utilization would be high at first and that providers might absorb some early losses. It was hoped that the participants would find the plan so attractive and would be so satisfied with it that they would sign up for subsequent years—when they wouldn't require services—and the providers could make up any losses from the first years by enjoying the capitation rate without having to provide services. The trend today is towards contracts with longer duration periods. Most plan administrators are looking for contracts that last two or three years, thereby ensuring that providers could profit. The hope that participants would continue in the plan on their own simply didn't materialize. They didn't renew the contracts with the alacrity predicted by administrators.

The problem here is with marketing. It is much easier to entice a group into trying a plan for a one-year period, than it is to get them to commit to something that lasts three years. In addition, if you find that you have incorporated some things into the plan that you don't really like, you are stuck with them as well. It is a two-sided coin. The best advice is to plan well, and try for a longer contract. You can negotiate it down from there if necessary. Regardless, you will have to incorporate something into the contract that points out to members that they must remain in the plan for a specified period. Remember to make sure that the time period corresponds with that specified in your provider contract so that you will still have providers for the entire period of the subscriber contract. You might have a clause like this:

> Plan Enrollees shall agree to remain in the plan for a period of one (1) year from the date the Enrollee's coverage begins, or until such time as the Enrollee becomes ineligible, whichever first occurs.

Termination and Continuation

Capitation contracts should provide for releases in the event things change. Failure on the part of master subscribers to pay the bill is a good example. But before you design this part of the contract, go back and read your provider contract. Just as with the clause on the duration of the contract, it is important to weave the same threads of logic through this section to ensure that DMI is able to fulfill its obligations and provide an escape in the event that it isn't.

> **Termination.** Termination of Contracted Dental Services shall occur under the following conditions:
>
> 1. Contracted dental services for any Enrollee shall automatically terminate on the first day of the month following:
>
>   a. Termination of this agreement for any reason provided herein.

b. Amendment of this agreement so as to terminate the services available for the class of Enrollees for which said Enrollees are members.

c. The failure of an Enrollee to pay any premium required to be paid within the time period allowable.

d. Termination of employment or association membership with the Master Subscriber.

2. Dependent services available for any dependent of an Enrollee shall terminate on the first day of the month following the date the person ceases to be a dependent as defined, or, if earlier, upon the termination of the services available for the Enrollee, or upon failure to pay any premium required for such services within the time period allowable.

3. If, after reasonable efforts, the Provider is unable to establish and maintain a satisfactory dentist-patient relationship with an Enrollee and/or dependents, the plan may be terminated by DMI without further obligation of either party to the other, except for payment of any money which may then be due.

4. In the event that DMI is unable, by using its best efforts, to obtain the services of Providers and their staffs to render the Contracted Dental Services to Enrollees, under this agreement, for a period of thirty (30) days after the date upon which such services first became unavailable, then and in that event, this agreement shall terminate without further obligation of any of the parties to the other, or to any Enrollee or Eligible Dependent entitled to services thereunder, except for the payment of any money which may then be due.

5. In the event that performance of the terms and conditions of this agreement, or any agreement which DMI has with a Provider in connection therewith is rendered invalid or impossible by act of governmental authority, this agreement shall terminate without further obligation of either party to the other, or to any Enrollee or Eligible Dependent entitled to services hereunder, except for the payment of any money which may then be due, whether by refund of prepaid but unearned dental services or otherwise. Further, and in any event, DMI may terminate this Agreement without cause by sixty (60) days written notice to the applicable Master Subscriber without obligation except as hereinabove provided.

Continuation. This Agreement shall be continued in force by payment of the premium as set forth herein.

Capitation Rate

This part of the contract is perhaps the most important from the standpoint of DMI's financial aspirations. It is critical to spell out exactly who will pay and how much they are responsible for. What happens with rate changes and changes in the number of enrollees should also be addressed. You will have to custom design this part of the agreement to fit exactly the set of circumstances for which you have contracted. Some general principles are included in the contract to aid you in customizing.

You may find that a master subscriber is interested in paying only part of the capitation rate and intends to have the members pay the rest. You will want to account for it in this part of the contract, but if possible, try to get him to pay it all and collect the rest from employees. Basically, the amount due on any due date by each master subscriber is determined by the premium charge in effect on any date times the number of persons then enrolled for services. In addition to the monthly capitation rate, you may be able to charge a one-time administration fee to the master subscriber. Many companies are able to charge this extra fee which can be used to off-set some of the marketing costs. Master subscribers sometimes balk about this, especially since it is they who are actually keeping track of employees and rates. It probably isn't worth alienating the client, but if you can get it, be sure to specify in the contract that it is to be paid. Be sure to leave yourself some room to change the rates later if you find that it is difficult to make it on the rate you have agreed to.

Capitation Payments. The following terms are agreed to regarding capitation payments:

1. The Master Subscriber shall pay to DMI a monthly charge of _____ per single Enrollee and ____per family.
2. The Master Subscriber shall pay an initial yearly administration fee of: ____.
3. The initial monthly rate times the number of Enrollees shall be paid each month during the term of this Agreement until changed and shall not be changed for the first Contract Year as that term is defined in the master contract. DMI reserves the right to establish new

monthly rates on any due date after the first Contract Year upon thirty (30) days notice to the Master Subscriber.

4. The amount due on any due date by each Master Subscriber shall be determined by the premium charge in effect on such date and the persons then enrolled for services.

5. By separate agreement attached hereto as Addendum "A" between DMI and the Master Subscriber, capitation rates may be payable other than monthly. If the charges are payable other than monthly and any change in the number of plan Enrollees occurs within the period, a pro rata adjustment of the charges shall be computed from the first day of the Contract Month coincident with or next following the date such change occurs, and the total capitation rate for the payment period shall be as adjusted.

6. If the amount paid for any period is less than the amount due, the Master Subscriber shall pay the balance to DMI at the termination of such period. If amount paid is greater than amount due, DMI shall then return the excess to the Master Subscriber.

7. All capitation rates are payable by each Master Subscriber in advance to DMI by mail at the address listed in this Agreement, or at such other address that DMI may designate in writing. If any charge is not paid by the Master Subscriber when due, then this Agreement may be terminated by DMI except as provided herein.

8. If prior to the due date of any premium charge after the first contract month, a Contract Agreement has not been terminated for any reason as set forth herein, and DMI has not then given notice of its refusal to continue such Contract Agreement, a grace period of one (l) month from the date any payment is due will be granted for the payment of such premium charge, during which time such Contract Agreement shall remain in force. If a Master Subscriber fails to pay within the grace period, its Contract Agreement shall automatically terminate at the expiration of the grace period and such Master Subscriber shall be liable to DMI for the payment of all amounts then due and unpaid including the prepaid charge for the grace period.

With a generic agreement such as this, when the sign-up drive is completed, DMI will merely have to send a billing to the master subscriber for the first month premium. From a tactical standpoint it would not be a bad idea to send a bill each month after the master subscriber indicates any changes in his number of enrollees. The contract assumes automatic payment, but the cost of actually sending the bill out each month by DMI is far outweighed by the increased response.

Co-payments

This contract is actually between the master subscriber and the capitation company. Co-payments are between the patients and the providers. Nevertheless, policies regarding them should be clearly spelled out in this agreement. Presumably the agreement will be available to individual members; in any case, the co-payment policies should be outlined. Some possible wording for the co-pay section of the agreement might be as follows:

Co-payments. The following conditions shall be agreed to regarding co-payments:

1. Co-payment Services shall be available to Enrollees and dependents on a voluntary basis. Each Enrollee electing such services shall advise the Provider of such election.
2. Any participation in Co-payment Services elected by an Enrollee will terminate if eligibility of said Enrollee is terminated according to the provisions of this agreement or if this Master Subscriber Agreement is terminated.
3. All charges for Co-payment Services shall be paid by the Enrollee directly to the Provider rendering such services. Payments will be made at the time of delivery of the services.
4. In the event of termination of this contract, or termination of the contract between DMI and the provider, or loss of eligibility of the Member, the Dentist shall be responsible to complete work started prior to the termination of said contract or contracts, as follows:
   a. If an impression has been taken, the dentist shall complete a denture or partial.
   b. The Dentist shall complete work which may have been started on any individual tooth.

Out of Area Treatment

The HMO Act states that a member of a capitation plan may be entitled to reimbursement for expenses incurred for treatments rendered by other than the organization in the case where the treatments were "medically necessary and immediately required." Most dental prepaid programs include some sort of benefit to enrollees for treatment delivered out of the immediate area of service, as for example, when one of your members is on vacation and requires emergency treatment.

A few caveats apply here. First of all, in your contract you should specify an exact distance away from one of your offices to constitute "out of area." If you don't, a patient may just go to any dentist and say his or her treatment was an emergency, and you will have to pay for it. Fifty miles is not an unreasonable distance to set for this requirement. If someone is within that distance, it would not be unreasonable for you to expect them to visit one of the offices in your system. In a very rural area you may want to increase that distance. People in the country are used to traveling for services.

Additionally, remember, it is the capitation company that is responsible for paying for the service delivered out of area; therefore you will want to set some limitations on the amount and on the type of service to be delivered. This concept is intended to provide some sort of emergency treatment. You do not want patients to be able to have a crown done on their trip to Maui and send you the bill. Wording for this part of the contract might go like this:

Out of Area Treatment. Such treatment shall be covered as follows:

1. Should an Enrollee require emergency dental treatment while outside of an area of fifty (50) miles from his/her dental facility, the plan will cover reimbursement of dental charges incurred for necessary treatment in the case of the following:
   a. Control of bleeding
   b. Control of infection
   c. Relief of pain associated with dental problems
2. Any procedures in excess of alleviating the immediate emergency will not be reimbursed under the plan. In any event, the maximum allowable charge for any one occurrence will not exceed fifty dollars ($50.00). Additional procedures required must be done at the Enrollee's regular DMI dental facility.

General Provisions

The balance of the contract contains general provisions of the plan. Check back with your provider contract to see if you have incorporated any additional provisions which should be followed through in this subscriber agreement. Some of these general provisions, like the workmen's compensation clause, are outlined by the HMO Act. Others such as the Information Required clause are included as a matter of logistics and administrative ease.

Independent Nature of Provider. It is understood and agreed that any individual engaged to perform Provider Services shall be independent, and not employees of, nor under the control, supervision, or management of DMI and that DMI shall not be liable to any Master Subscriber or any Enrollee for any negligent, willful, or wrongful act or omission of whatever nature, performed by any individual engaged to perform Provider Services hereunder or by a member of such individual's staff.

Legal Actions. No action at law or in equity shall be brought to recover on any Contract Agreement prior to the expiration of sixty (60) days after written notice has been furnished to DMI specifying the grounds for such action.

Appointments. Priorities in scheduling appointments shall be as follows:

1. Emergency care
2. First time visits for examination and treatment
3. Regular non-emergency dental care

Any Enrollee (including a dependent) who fails to keep an appointment shall be subject to a _______ charge by the Provider unless the appointment is cancelled at least twenty-four (24) hours prior to the scheduled appointment and such charge shall be paid by the Enrollee directly to the Provider.

Information Required. Each Master Subscriber shall furnish to DMI all information which DMI may reasonably require with regard to matters pertaining to the services afforded by this agreement. All documents, books, and records which may have a bearing on such services, any participation in this plan, or charges under such agreement shall be open for inspection by DMI at all reasonable times during the continuance of such Contract Agreement and within one (1) year after its final termination.

Eligibility information will include, but shall not be limited to, the name and address of each Enrollee and Eligible Dependent. Each Master Subscriber shall supply on a monthly basis records to update the list of Eligible Members and Eligible Dependents. The Master Subscriber shall not include any person on the list of Enrollees if not eligible.

Conformity with State Statutes. The laws of the State of __________ shall govern, and be used for the interpretation, construction, and enforcement of this Agreement. Any provision thereof which is in conflict with the statutes or applicable regulations of the State will be amended to conform to the minimum requirements or regulations, provided that DMI in its sole and absolute discretion, determines that conforming with such statutes or regulations shall be possible.

Effect on Worker's Compensation. This agreement does not fulfill any requirement of worker's compensation or other compulsory insurance and cannot be used in lieu thereof.

Pre-existing Conditions. Services as described under thisAgreement shall be delivered to Enrollees regardless of the date of inception of the dental defect for which treatment is required.

Notices. Any notice, consent, or other communication required by, or to be given pursuant to this Agreement shall be in writing and delivered to the intended recipient thereof. A writing shall be deemed delivered if mailed to the intended recipient by certified mail, return receipt requested, postage prepaid.

Third Party Rights. All rights and liabilities created under this Agreement shall be deemed to exist only as between DMI and the Master Subscriber. In no event shall this Agreement be deemed to confer any right on or create any obligation to any third party not a signatory or to create in such third party a status of third party beneficiary.

Addendum. Any addendum signed by DMI and a Master Subscriber as part of this Agreement shall constitute a part of this Agreement as if such additional provision were originally set forth. However, any provision in such addendum that is contrary to or inconsistent with any of the original provisions shall prevail over and supersede such original contrary or inconsistent provision.

Assignment. This Agreement shall bind and inure to the benefit of the parties hereto, their respective heirs, personal representatives, successors and assigns. This Agreement and any rights or obigations relating thereto may not be assigned by the Master Subscriber without the prior written consent of DMI, which consent shall not be reasonably withheld.

Nontransferability. Contract dental services provided under this plan are personal to Enrollees and are not assignable.

Specific Provider. All dental services are to be provided to Enrollee by the specific Provider chosen by the Enrollee at the time of enrollment as designated on the enrollment application. An Enrollee may upon written notice to DMI change to a different Provider. Such change is to be effective the first day of the month following such written notification.

Dental Review Panel. DMI shall appoint a Dental Review Panel, made up of licensed dentists who shall advise and assist DMI in the supervision of standards of dental care, matters which relate to the dentist-patient relationship, methods and manners of operation, costs and necessity of treatment. The decision of the Dental Review Panel shall be binding on all parties hereto.

Finally, under the general provision part of the agreement, it might be wise to incorporate some wording that refers to whatever decision you have made regarding specialty referrals. Enrollees should be advised that they must visit specialists in the plan or pay for services themselves. It might read like this:

Specialty Referral. DMI shall furnish to each of its Providers a list of specialists under contract to DMI to provide services to Enrollees. Members requiring the services of a specialist must visit one of the specialists on the list. If a member elects to seek the services of a specialist not on the list or if DMI does not have an available specialist for the services in an Enrollee's area, then the Enrollee must pay for the services of said specialist directly. No benefits under this plan will be granted to Enrollees seeking specialty treatment from specialists other than those under contract to DMI.

Coordination of Benefits

Since your first plan will probably be a basic services plan, when you offer it initially to small groups it is not very likely that you will find many members signing up who are covered by additional indemnifying insurance coverage. It simply would not be worth it to them. Later as you begin to diversify your presentations, it may become a possibility. Nonetheless, you should decide in the beginning whether you intend to offer your clients a primary plan or a secondary plan.

If a capitation plan is offered as the primary plan, only the charges for the co-payments can be charged to the indemnifying carrier for payment. If the capitation plan is offered as the secondary plan, then the entire fee-for-service charge fee can be billed to the indemnifying carrier. If their payment exceeds the amount of the co-payment, then the dentist involved can keep the overpayment. If the payment from the indemnifier is less than the co-payment, then the patient is responsible for the difference.

Since the co-payment is usually significantly low, it is to your advantage to offer your plan as a secondary plan. Some states may have regulations regarding primary and secondary coverage, so check on these first. Be sure your contract tells patients which type your plan is, but don't worry too much about it because if you are starting small and offering a basic coverage plan to those groups who have nothing else, it will not come up very often.

> **Coordination of Benefits.** The DMI Plan shall be considered as the secondary plan should such DMI Enrollee possess any other dental benefit plan. The other dental benefit coverage an Enrollee may have will be assigned to the Provider performing the Contracted Dental Services and will be considered as "primary" coverage in the order of determining dental plan benefits.

Exclusions

The subscriber contract ends with the same list of exclusions as the provider contract. Each exclusion is relatively self-explanatory when you think in terms of greater profits if less treatment is performed. Pick and choose the ones that seem important to you. But remember, if you rule everything out, your credibility will suffer and that is a major concern. Remember too that capitation plans have failed because of too much profit-oriented thinking on the part of the providers and plan administrators. The secret for success is to give the patients quality, affordable service. They expect and deserve it. They may not realize when you are providing that type of service, but they will certainly know when you are not!

Exclusions. This plan does not include the following:

1. Visits to or services performed by a specialist, dentist, or provider not part of the provider
2. Any dental services which are necessitated as a result of war or any act of war whether such war be declared or undeclared, riot, insurrection, or civil disturbance
3. Any dental services arising out of any sickness or injury arising out of or sustained in the course of any occupation or employment for remuneration or profit
4. Any dental services which, in the judgment of the Dentist, are not reasonable and necessary for the prevention, correction, or im- provement of a condition
5. Any dental services not specifically described in the Schedule of Benefits (including hospital charges or prescription drug charges)
6. Any dental services which are necessitated as a result of a self-inflicted condition
7. Any dental services for which the Enrollee is reimbursed, entitled to reimbursement, or is in any way indemnified for such expenses by or through any public program, state or federal, or any program of medical or dental benefits sponsored and paid for by the Federal Government or any agency thereof
8. Any dental services necessitated as a result of a condition sustained in the commission of or the attempt to commit a felony
9. Oral surgery requiring the setting of fractures or dislocations
10. Treatment of malignancies, cysts, or neoplasms
11. Dispensing of drugs for treatment of oral disease not normally supplied in a dental office
12. Congenital defects

13. Conditions affecting the temporomandibular joint including dysfunction and/or malocclusion
14. Any costs or expenses incurred in the event the Enrollee is hospitalized for any dental procedure
15. Services of an anesthetist or anesthesiologist
16. Gold or gold foil restorations
17. Any dental charges incurred for treatment of obesity
18. Appliances or restoration necessary to increase vertical dimension or to restore an occlusion
19. Programs or treatment which were in progress prior to the date any person became an Enrollee under this plan
20. Any new services or procedures performed after the last day of the month during which any person ceased to be eligible for participation under this plan
21. Services which are of a such complexity that they cannot be performed by the contracted Providers within the plan

Closing

Finally, our contract should spell out the effective date and duration of the agreement, close, and provide for signatures of executives representing the master subscriber and DMI. Be sure to set the effective date far enough ahead to handle administrative details such as marketing to individual members and open enrollment.

This Agreement shall be effective the ____ day of __________ ,19 ___ , and shall be continued thereafter for a period of one (1) year unless terminated according to the terms herein.

This Agreement contains the entire agreement, understanding and all representations and warranties between the parties hereto. No change in this Agreement shall be valid unless approved by an executive officer of DENTAL MAINTENANCE INTERNATIONAL, INC. and an executive of the company.

IN WITNESS WHEREOF, the parties have caused this Agreement to be executed as of the date mentioned above.

Master Subscriber	**DMI**
by: ____________	**by:** ____________
Address ____________	Address ____________
City/State ____________	City/State ____________
ZIP Code ____________	ZIP Code ____________
Phone ____________	Phone ____________

Fee Schedule

The contract is not really complete until we provide both the master subscriber and the potential enrollees a copy of the co-payment fees that they will be charged. It should be attached to the contract as Addendum "A." A copy of a sample fee schedule is included in Appendix B of this book, by way of example only. The fees are in no way representative of current fees in any plan. Their inclusion is to demonstrate which fees are frequently associated with co-pays and which are not. Your schedule may differ dramatically.

Remember to view this discussion of subscriber contracts as an example only. Your lawyer may suggest the inclusion of additional points to satisfy conditions in your state or specific conditions of the plan you develop for a particular group. The number of legal clauses that may apply to dental capitation contracts is limitless.

Chapter 8 Marketing the Product

Now that we have developed our capitation product, made it legal, provided for sound relations with the dentists who will actually deliver the services, and established the basics of a plan for dealing with subscribers, we must begin to sell the plan to groups. This, as with all business ventures, is of critical importance.

Defining Groups

The first rule to selling anything is "Know your product." The second is "Know your market." Our market is the groups of people who will eventually become actual patients. To break this down farther, the basic group is simply an individual with no ties to any particular employer or organization. Next is the family of that individual. From that basic group we can move up the scale to an individual who is linked to an employer of some sort. Next is his family, and then come groups of families linked by a common employer. From there, we can move to individuals and families who are members of an association, and finally groups linked by a common union or trust fund.

Without any question, the most difficult of these potential clients to deal with is the single individual. The major reason? The individual who independently elects to choose a capitation dental plan expects to be a heavy utilizer. Unquestionably, in this case, costs of treatment will leap far ahead of revenue collected. Unless the contract is long enough to allow premiums to catch up with costs, the provider of services to this individual will find it difficult to break even. In addition, collections from individuals are much harder to make. Unless you have received the entire premium payment in one lump at the beginning of the contract period, you may find it difficult to collect payments on a regular basis. The concept of "prepaid plan" is strained a bit under these circumstances.

At the other end of the spectrum is the employer/employee group. It is here that prepaid dentistry has made the biggest advances. If the group is small enough, you may run into the same problems as with individuals. As the numbers of potential clients in a particular group rise, the chances of heavy utilization drop. In any group, you will have individuals who do not require treatment, some who will not seek it, and some who will wait too long and allow the contract to expire before services are requested. This allows providers the opportunity to collect some reserves before incurring costs. If an employer is sending one check to your capitation company for many individuals or families, collection problems will be dramatically decreased.

Somewhere between these extremes lie the associations. We can divide them into two groups. First are associations which have no financial strings attached to their members. At least, financial requirements for membership (such as dues) do not cover particular member services like health care. Other associations, secondly, are based on existing or previous monetary attachments. Unions and members represented by trust funds are examples. Dealing with the first type of associations (which we could call "clubs") is similar to dealing with individuals. Indeed, what you will end up having, if the association is not paying the premiums, is a group of individual contracts. If you are accepting payments periodically instead of single lump payments, you will have all of the collection headaches that come with that arrangement. Usually when you are accepting payments from associations which can write one check for all members who have elected participation in the plan, these worries are eliminated. Utilization problems with members of associations who are paying their own premiums parallel those of individuals in general.

Marketing for individuals and for groups can be dramatically different for capitation companies. If you are marketing strictly to individuals, all of the related expenses, from postage to proposals, will be borne by your company. If you are marketing to an employer/employee, you may be able to obtain some assistance. You may be able to get the employer to send one of your marketing packages to his employees. He may even bear the cost of having the package produced. Or, he may be willing to have a special meeting of all of his employees who are interested where you can solicit them via an explanatory lecture. He may have an employee newsletter, or may allow you to place association letter in employee pay vouchers. At the very least, he will be able to provide you with names and addresses which will eliminate some of the shotgun marketing necessary when dealing with individuals. Some employers have been willing to follow all of these suggestions including the development of elaborate brochures. This is where negotiating skills are important.

If you work with associations, you may find a mixed degree of cooperation. Some may be able to do nothing other than provide you with a list of names. If you are lucky, you may be able to entice them into providing you with mailing labels if they have computer capabilities. Others may go to the same extent as some employer/employee groups by providing printed materials or articles in newsletters. You will not know until you begin to research the particular organization.

Oversubscribing

We have said that one thing that will kill your capitation plan is the delivery of inferior services. Another lethal mistake is oversubscription. The tendency when beginning to offer capitation plans to groups is to succumb to visions of big money. The thought that ten employees in a group generate X dollars, and therefore a 100-employee group will generate ten times as much, is tempting. If however, individual enrollees in your plan are unable to obtain an appointment to see one of the providers, they quickly will become disenchanted. Your credibility will be bruised, and you will find that enrollees are reluctant to re-sign their contracts in the profitable later years of the plan.

Think about that when you are considering groups. If it is a larger group, will it be necessary to gear up to handle them or can they be worked easily into the existing schedule? Will you need additional providers to handle them? Will the demand additional providers if your offices are too small, or not located conveniently for the majority of their members? You may find that they are thinking about these things and you should be as well. And remember, just because a group of people place their mobile homes in the same park, that does not necessarily mean they will be a good group. It is important that they are linked by a stronger bond, or administrative hassles can get out of control.

To be on the safe side, let's assume that DMI plans has chosen the conservative route and is hoping to sign up those employer/employee groups with 2–50 members first. They intend to approach them one at a time, and only after they are worked adequately into the schedule will they add groups to the plan.

Word of Mouth

The first thing DMI will have to do in order to enroll some members in the plan is to attract some attention. The best way of course is by word of mouth. If you are offering the plan directly out of your office or are in a group of providers who want to offer plans for your collective offices, talk to some of your patients. It will not be difficult to find someone without dental insurance who is willing to listen. As a matter of fact, if you have a motivated listener, you may find that they are willing to do most of the marketing for you as well. Many people working in small companies without coverage know their fellow employees very well. They may be willing to talk to some of them for you and with their help and pressure, you may find it easier to approach their employer with a prospective plan. This will be even easier if the employees are willing to pay for it themselves at first, until you can get it flowing for awhile. Finding the right person is critical. Some may nod, and say "Sounds good," but never do anything. Others may want the specifics of the plan that day because they are on their way to visit with fellow workers to convince them to join the plan. If you are fortunate enough to find an employer in your chair who has been considering some sort of plan for his workers (as well as himself), so much the better. Negotiations can proceed immediately.

Solicitation Letter

If word of mouth isn't working, you will have to resort to the next best thing. If you have a lot of money, that would be television commercials, but if not, a simple solicitation letter may do the trick. Canvas the telephone book, and call the chamber of commerce. Prepare a list of potential businesses in your area that employ the number of people that seems right for your provider list. Call them on the phone and ask the first secretary who answers if the company has dental insurance. If they do not, move them to the top of the list, and send them a letter. Try to send it to the chief officer of the company at first. The personal touch is always better than a generic letter that might as well be written from one computer to another. That is not to say that you cannot use your computer. You purchased it to use it for this kind of job. Make up a letter and have the computer change the names and addresses for multiple delivery.

Make the letter brief and to the point. One page is usually adequate. If they are interested, they will respond. If the letter is too long, they will not even finish it. Try to make the letter as interesting as possible but don't over do it. You don't want to sound like a carnival barker. An example of a solicitation letter might be as follows:

DENTAL MAINTENANCE INTERNATIONAL
2972 Elm Street
Maple, Michigan 48888

John J. Jones
Jones Industries, Inc.
P.O. Box 555
Maple, MI 48888

Dear Mr. Jones,

Good news! Dental Maintenance International is offering selected businesses in Maple an opportunity to participate in a program that could, **without cost,** add a dental plan to existing employee benefit packages. That's right. Now you can provide dental coverage for your employees at absolutely no cost to you. Of course, if you would like to contribute to the plan, that option is always open, and flexible, so that you can determine exactly how you will use the plan.

Sound interesting? Dental Maintenance International is administering these plans in your area with the help of some very well respected dentists, such as Dr. __________ . We are happy to say the plans have been very successful! Our plans have met with the specifications required by the state and we have been granted a certificate of authority under public act __________________________.

Our programs are strictly voluntary. Only those employees who wish to participate are invited to join. There are no minimum subscriber numbers before the plan is operational. This helps to assure that people who do not need services do not end up paying for those who do!

To outline the plan briefly: Participants pay a small monthly fee, which then entitles them to receive dental treatment at fees far below industry norms whenever they visit a participating DMI dental office. It couldn't be simpler! Premium rates vary, depending on the size of the group, but we are certain your employees will find them attractive at any level.

You will be happy to know, this plan:

1. Has no troublesome claim forms
2. Covers pre-existing conditions
3. Has no yearly maximums

And, let me repeat: Your financial participation is not necessary!

I would like the opportunity to meet with you to answer any questions you may have and to explain the program to you in greater detail. If you are interested, please contact me at Dental Maintenance International (555-4323).

Kindest regards,

Dental Maintenance International

The wording in this letter may not be exactly correct for you, but the general format should get you thinking about customizing it. You may not want to (or be in a position to) include the name of a specific doctor in the letter, but if you can use a name to help ensure credibility, it could be valuable.

If the letter approach does not work, try another one. Some advertisements simply come across better than others, and that is exactly what this is. If it still doesn't work, try sending it to individuals you know who work at that particular business. If they become interested, they may be able to influence their employer at least to listen to you. Always remember to follow up the letter with a phone call to see if you can answer any questions the employer may have.

Conventional Marketing

While we are seeing more and more advertisements by dentists in the conventional manner, i.e., media advertising as well as direct and internal marketing, some dentists may be still uncomfortable with the idea. Old notions of professionalism are difficult to change. Many feel that dentistry is still an art and a science, and should reside on a plateau above the used car and appliance businesses, where media marketing has reached new lows. The results of such advertising, however, are nonetheless desired by those same practitioners. They are looking for new business just as the conventional advertisers are. Since the capitation company is an entity at least one step removed from the dentist, it can offer a new opportunity to benefit from some form of conventional advertising. The capitation company can produce advertisements in the newspapers, on the radio, and even on television, and maintain a blanket of insulation for the dentist. There is nothing wrong with hiring some professional advertisers to help you to sell your programs. If you can work it into your budget, you may find this to be an excellent way of gaining clients for you, and new patients for the dentists in your plan.

Plan Proposal

When you receive a response to one of your marketing methods, you will have to set up a meeting to explain the entire program. To make the sales meeting run smoothly, and to make sure that the results are in your favor, you will want to control the situation. The best way to handle this is to present a detailed plan proposal, in writing, that those present can follow and refer to. You should present this proposal to each of the members who will attend the meeting, preferably in advance. Your computer can store them for you and you can simply change the various names and pertinent clauses, or add an addendum or two to satisfy criteria for the specific group. Be sure to take extra copies to the meeting to distribute to others who may be present.

In many cases, you will not be able to set up a personal meeting and your written plan proposal is the only sales device you will have. Some larger groups simply "take bids and proposals" and you may never have the opportunity to do much explaining. Therefore your plan proposal should outline the highlights of your plan in a concise and professional manner. It should only sound like a sales pitch to the extent that it should provoke further interest on the part of the prospective clients. Watch your credibility here. The proposal should contain copies of the subscriber contract as well as lists of providers and co-pay fees. It should, of course, contain the capitation rate you intend to charge. Be careful not to make the didactic part too long, or no one will read it. Merely outline the highlights of the plan. A typical plan proposal might look something like this:

Dental Maintenance International
Prepaid Dental Plans

Plan Proposal

The DMI group prepaid dental plan is designed for employer-employee groups, unions, associations, or membership groups. The plan benefits and requirements are outlined below.

GROUP SIZE REQUIREMENT: There is a minimum of three (3) participants needed to institute the DMI Dental Plan.

This plan may be offered as a voluntary benefit with no sponsor contribution required.

PLAN BENEFITS: Eligible plan participants pay a monthly premium either directly or through payroll deductions which entitles them and their eligible dependents to a comprehensive collection of dental benefits.

The DMI Group Prepaid Dental Plan provides 100% coverage for basic routine dental services. These include treatment for diagnostic, preventative, routine restorative and routine oral surgery. A complete list of benefits and allowances is attached as Exhibit A.

For those services which require specialized procedures, there is a co-payment.

THERE ARE:

No Deductibles

Unlimited Maximums

No Claim Forms to Complete

No Denial of Coverage for Pre-existing Conditions

AVAILABILITY OF BENEFITS: To receive benefits, participants must visit authorized DMI participating dental offices. A list of these offices is attached as Exhibit B.

ELIGIBILITY: Employees of Employer Groups and Members of Unions, Associations or Membership Groups and their children from birth to age 19, or to age 23 if unmarried and attending an accredited educational institution on a full-time basis, may apply for benefits under this plan.

PLAN EFFECTIVE DATE: Plans may be made effective only on the first day of the month. Participants may begin services on the effective date. There is no waiting period for any available services once a participant's plan becomes effective.

OPEN ENROLLMENT PERIODS: Participants are only to enter the plan at the time they are initially eligible, or at the time of open enrollment. Open Enrollments will be held once a year on the contract anniversary date.

PARTICIPATION: An eligible member may join the Prepaid Dental Plan on the initial effective date of the plan or, for new participants, after a waiting period designated by the Group. After enrollment, the participant must remain in the plan for a period of one year, or as long as such participant is still considered eligible for benefits under the plan.

OUT OF AREA TREATMENT: Should a participant have an emergency situation occur outside an area of 50 miles or more from where his/her dental facility is located, the plan will provide coverage for:

1. Control of bleeding
2. Control of infection
3. Relief of pain associated with dental problems

Itemized charges for these coverage should be presented to the DMI Home Office or the Prepaid Group Dental Facility. The maximum allowable charge will be $50.

If it is necessary to have additional treatment, it must be provided at the Prepaid Group Dental Facility.

TERMINATION: Upon termination of eligibility of a participant, the Plan benefits will extend to the end of the month in which termination occurs. Procedures in progress at termination will be completed.

Exclusions and Limitations

The following are not covered under the Plan:

1. Visits to or services performed by a specialist or dentist not part of the Prepaid Dental Group
2. Sickness or injury arising out of or sustained in the course of any occupation or employment for remuneration or profit

3. Reimbursement of cost: (Dental Groups will bill any additional charges to the participant. These charges will not be reimbursed by DMI.)
4. Any dental services which, in the judgment of the Prepaid Dental Group are not reasonable and necessary for the prevention, correction, or improvement of a condition
5. Dental Services not specifically described in the Schedule of Benefits
6. Any service deemed too difficult for our prepaid providers to do effectively

THE DMI DENTAL PLAN MAY BE PURCHASED FOR AS LITTLE AS:

Single Participant	**$** ________________
Dependents	**$** ________________
Family	**$** ________________
Flat Group Monthly Administration Fee	**$** ________________

RATES ARE FIRM AND GUARANTEED FOR A PERIOD OF ONE YEAR FROM THE EFFECTIVE DATE OF THE PLAN REGARDLESS OF ACTUAL ENROLLMENT.

This proposal expires on ________________________

Sign-up Drive

If the board of directors of the group you are soliciting decides to accept your plan, you will next have to market it to his employees and sign them into the plan. As we have discussed, try to use the employer to assist in this as much as possible. Use his pay envelopes, and any newsletters he may already have. If it is a small company, try to set up a meeting with the employees. Make a presentation to them outlining the points you and the employer have agreed to and then have a question-and-answer period.

At the very least, try to get the employer to send his employees a letter, which you will design, using his stationery.

Announcement Letter

Ultimately you will have to devise some sort of introductory letter which announces the existence of your agreement. If you can, try to get the employer to send this letter to his employees. Design it yourself and handle all of the actual mailing, but use his stationery. An example using Fred's Tool and Die as an employer might read like this:

Fred's Tool and Die
24 State Street
Maple, Michigan 48888

Date

Dear Fred's Employee,

Good news! Fred's Tool and Die has entered into an agreement with DENTAL MAINTENANCE INTERNATIONAL to provide a COMPREHENSIVE PREPAID DENTAL PROGRAM for you! Your membership in our group of employees will entitle you and your family to receive top quality dental health care at prices far below the industry norms. You will be happy to know that this plan:

- Has no troublesome claim forms
- Has no deductibles
- Has no yearly maximums
- Covers pre-existing conditions

Sound interesting? A brochure available at the personnel office outlines the highlights of the Dental Maintenance International prepaid dental program and includes a list of any co-payment fees you may have to pay for services when you visit one of the prepaid facilities. In order to receive benefits under the Dental Maintenance International program, you must visit one of our prepaid facilities listed in the brochure.

Participation in this program is strictly voluntary. If you would like to join, complete the 3 X 5 application card available at the personnel office and return it to: Dental Maintenance International, 2972 Elm, Maple, MI 48888. All applications must be received by , so do not hesitate.

Applicants to the Dental Maintenance International prepaid dental program agree to remain in the plan for one year and to pay a monthly premium of:

One Person

Family (2 or more)

This premium will be taken from your pay automatically if you desire to participate in the plan.

The Fred's Tool and Die Board of Directors would like to encourage all of our employees to take advantage of this program. If you have any questions, please inquire at the personnel office or call Dental Maintenance International at 555-1111.

Sincerely,

Fred's Tool and Die

Member Packet or Brochure

In addition to the announcement letter, you will have to design an information packet for the individual employees who sign up. This packet must point out the salient features of the master subscriber contract and should remind employees of a few key points:

1. They must remain in the plan for the entire period of the contract as specified in the master subscriber agreement.
2. They must sign up for and visit a specific dental office in the plan.
3. Treatment will only be available at that office.
4. Co-payments must be paid directly to the providers at the time of service.
5. Certain procedures are excluded from the plan.
6. Your specialist arrangements should be explained.
7. The method you have chosen for payment of premiums— direct or payroll deductions should be clearly stated.

A good method for accomplishing this task, and one that will help to bolster that all-important credibility, is to design a professional-looking brochure that outlines the plan. Get together with a reputable printer and be prepared to spend some time on it. Be sure that it serves the dual purpose of explaining the details of the plan and markets it as well. Be sure to list all of the offices where dental treatment will be available, and include a list of the co-pay fees. These lists can be printed on a single sheet that folds into the brochure so that it can be replaced for updating without the necessity of changing the entire brochure.

Enrollment Application

One of the most important items in your membership packet is the application and sign-up card. It is the link between the master subscriber, the capitation company, the doctor, and the actual patient. In spite of its importance, with the aid of small print, it can actually be done using cards as small as 3 X 5 inches. That is not to say it has to be done in that small format; increasing the size to 5 X 8 or even to a full page will work just as well. The advantage to condensing it into a smaller size is financial. The form should be a multi-copy carbonless style. It should have at least three copies: one that is sent to the master subscriber, one that is returned to the enrollee when he is accepted into the plan, and another that is retained by the capitation company. This type of form can become expensive, so wasting space is a consideration.

The application should have a section for the usual name, rank, and serial number type of information. It should indicate who the master subscriber is if any, and include any employment numbers pertinent to the employee. Be sure to get the member's address and phone number. This is helpful in case you ever want to get in contact with an enrollee without having first to go through the master subscriber. It is of particular importance if you are dealing with members of an association who may be paying their own premiums.

Be sure to get the social security number and birth date of the enrollee and the birth dates of all dependents, so that you can verify identification and eligibility. If a child is over the cutoff age, you will want to obtain proof of their enrollment in an accredited school before you accept them for membership.

Below the information section should be some words that do the actual linking of parties. Their implied meaning should form a mini-contract binding the individual patients to the capitation company. If possible these words should be customized for the particular situation at hand. They might differ slightly depending upon whether you are dealing with an employer/employee group, an association, or whatever.

Finally, employers cannot deduct amounts from the paychecks of employees without the employees' written consent. Your membership application should have a section in which the enrollee authorizes his employer to make the necessary deductions specifically to pay for this program or whatever part of it ends up as his responsibility. Payroll deductions by the employer with a subsequent single check to the capitation company is a far superior method of premium collection than individual contributions on the part of separate subscribers.

An example of a possible enrollment application follows:

APPLICATION

Primary Subscriber ____________________ Soc. Sec. # ________________

SEX M F DOB __________________ Phone ____________________

Address ____

City ______________________________ County ____________________

State __________________________________ ZIP ____________________

Employer or Group ____

Spouse __________ Date of Birth ______________________________

Other dependents you wish to enroll:

Child __________________________________ Date of Birth ____________

Child __________________________________ Date of Birth ____________

Child __________________________________ Date of Birth ____________

Child __________________________________ Date of Birth ____________

I/we have read the terms of the Dental Maintenance International dental program as described by the participation brochure enclosed in this packet. We do hereby apply for membership in the plan. We understand the rules and regulations of the plan as defined in the master subscriber agreement and outlined in this brochure and agree to be bound by the terms and conditions of the plan as therein defined. We agree to pay Dental Maintenance International the monthly premium fee designated in the master subscriber agreement upon acceptance into the plan, and to pay any and all additional fees directly to the providing dentists of the plan. We understand that services under this plan can only be received at participating Dental Maintenance International dental offices.

We agree to visit the dental office of ______________________
as listed in the Participating Dental Offices list in this packet.

Member Signature: ______________________ Date __________

Spouse Signature: ______________________ Date __________

I/we do hereby authorize payroll deductions to pay the monthly premiums due Dental Maintenance International for this plan.

Primary Subscriber: ______________________ Date __________

Spouse: ______________________ Date __________

Finally, include a mailing envelope in your packet so that it will be easier for the members to send in their applications. You can obtain a business return rate permit from the post office to help. Or you can make it possible for the employees to return the application directly to the employer who will forward them in bulk to you.

Containing Your Own Costs

Place the brochure and co-pay schedules along with the announcement letter and the participation application in a nice envelope and mail it to each of the employees individually. That is the best way to ensure your credibility, but there is a basic problem—it's very expensive! Printers have minimum order requirements for producing fancy brochures and applications. You may have to hire graphic design and layout people to help set up your brochure if you are not creative in that field. Envelopes and postage can add up fast, even with bulk mailing capabilities. If you are marketing your plan to a small group of subscribers for a modest fee, you may find yourself in the red even if you have excellent acceptance by the group's members.

Do some initial planning in this regard. Investigate the costs of providing fancy professional brochures, and the costs associated with mailing them. Look at the premiums you intend to charge and calculate what the break-even point is. How many subscribers will have to sign up for the plan in order to cover the cost of your sign-up campaign? Does your target group have that many members? How many will actually sign up? You might be surprised and even depressed to learn that initial sign-ups for your plan will be much lower than you expect. Indeed, fewer than expected enrollments are a distressing aspect of this business as a whole.

One solution to this cost-containment problem is to use your faithful computer. Using your word processing program, you can create the letters with no problem. The machine will print them without complaint indefinitely, and for only a fraction of what it would cost to have it done by a professional printer. The brochure is nice, but you can accomplish the same result by printing all of the necessary information, including contracts, in numbered-page report format. You do not have to have a carbonless three-copy application either. You can print it with your machine and include it at the end of the information packet. Upon acceptance, you can copy only those applications received and return them to the enrollees and the master subscriber. That will prevent the additional costs of creating documents for people who may not need them.

You don't have to mail anything either. You can ask the employer to send your letters to his employees or to place them in their pay envelopes. You may have to reduce your one-time administrative fee to him or eliminate it altogether. Put a stack of the information packets in a central location within his operation (like the payroll office) and mention in the announcement letter that they can pick one up at that location. That will avoid the expense of mailing the packets, and you only will have to print them as the need arises, because only people interested in signing up for the plan will seek one. Some employers with copy machines may be willing to duplicate the information for any employees interested in the plan. Skip the return mailing envelope as well. Place that burden in the hands of the individuals who want the plan.

As you think about it more and become increasingly confident with computer technology, you may be able to think of even less expensive ways to market the plan. Weigh the benefits of increasing your credibility against the realities of finances and choose a course that seems appropriate.

Why a Specific Enrollment Period?

When you are signing up participants for your program, be sure to set a specific enrollment period. Make it a month or so. Why? Wouldn't it be more profitable to let as many people in as possible as often as possible and thereby collect more premiums? It is tempting, and after you have your drive, you will invariably find individuals who ask if they can sign up late. One of the problems with capitation programs in general, as we have pointed out before, is that they have a tendency to attract patients who need services—people who will be high utilizers. You want your plan to be something of value. You want people to think of it as an opportunity. You want to avoid encouraging the idea in clients that if they ever have a toothache or break the crown of a tooth it will be okay to sign up for the program then—"pay for it only if I need it" type of thinking. Encouraging utilization other than for preventive procedures can be economically unsound.

"Use it only when you need it" mentality can be damaging to your credibility as well. If people develop a casual attitude towards the program, it will be easy for them to forget about signing up again the next year. On the other hand, if they have been forced to suffer without coverage, or pay for necessary treatment themselves during a contract period while their friends have been enjoying the benefits of the program, they will be eager to sign up next year.

If you allow people to enter the plan at any time and have not made arrangements for this in both your master subscriber agreement and your provider agreements, you may find that you are dealing with people who in essence are not covered contractually. That can be risky. Allowing people into the plan at different times divides the groups and means that instead of one contract agreement covering one group of people, you will have one contract agreement covering two or more groups, thereby diluting its strength. Each will have its own effective date, and each will have its own premium payment schedule. That will definitely increase your management headaches.

One important task to be completed during the sign-up drive is to establish which providers will treat which patients. Since the capitation company pays a portion of the capitation fee for each patient to the specific office they sign up for, it is important to make that designation as soon as possible. Since providers may have to plan ahead in order to assume the risk of providing treatment as mandated by the HMO/capitation concept, we would like to keep the parameters used in that planning relatively constant. Multiple signups complicate those decisions.

That is not to say that you can't accept multiple sign-ups. Just be sure to weigh the consequences and determine if it is going to be worth it. Say for example you are dealing with a group of 100 families. During your first sign-up, only 15 agree to participate. You collect the premiums and everything seems to run smoothly. After others in the group have had a chance to speak with their comrades about the plan, interest in joining the plan begins to mount. Soon the master subscriber says he has an additional 50 families pestering him to join the plan. Premium income will jump dramatically. The providers in the system are not being strained. The master subscriber has been a good client and you would not want to alienate him. He is willing to sign an addendum covering the additional enrollees. Your computer doesn't care. It can handle a million subscribers all with different effective dates and variable payments. So why not? Let them in. The opportunity might be worth it.

If you do though, don't prorate premiums. Either charge the new clients the same amount as the old members and have their contract expire at the same time or charge them the same and let their contract run for the same length of time as the original one. If you prorate the premiums you will make your original clients angry and your credibility will be dented. In addition, you will encouraged another economically unsound idea. You will have told people it is all right to wait until the contract is half over to sign up, pay a lower rate, and rush to the providers demanding service before the contract date expires. As you may have guessed, your providers won't think much of that idea either.

Managing Records

When your sign-up drive is over, you should have a stack of completed applications to deal with. Now it's time to turn to the computer again. This time however, you can rest your word processing program for awhile and rely on your filing program. Computer people call these database programs. In essence they are used to manage the records of your clients, to bill them, and to keep track of variable effective dates and variable eligibility of dependents. You can do this without a computer, but in this age of electronic office helpers, it is difficult to imagine that you would want to.

If you are unfamiliar with computer programs, don't let database programs scare you. They really are not that difficult to use. Basically they consist of two parts or two functions. The first part is used to design the manner in which you will store the data, and the second part is actually entering and using the data in a useful manner. For our purposes, we will want to organize our data exactly as it is on our application form. All of the information on it will be necessary in our records. In addition, we will want to add some information that will be used for office purposes only. We will want to add a space on each record that indicates the effective date of the plan. That way we can sort all of our records to find those linked by the same contract date. We will want to be able to sort our records by the name of the master subscriber as well as the amount of premium due and paid. Finally we will want to be able to sort our records by date of birth so that with just a few key strokes we can figure out which dependents have attained an age when they will require their own contract.

This information is important for billing. In spite of the fact that our contract indicates that master subscribers will automatically send their payment each month, it is a very good idea to prepare to bill them just the same. Most filing programs have report-printing capabilities. A simple report can be designed to print a bill for an individual master subscriber which can be placed in an envelope and mailed. That function is particularly valuable when dealing with different master subscribers and different effective dates. As your business grows, you will be working with different groups and will be required to manage records for each of them and provide those different billings each month. If you are dealing with multiple individual contracts as will be the case if you contract with an association, you could be sending hundreds of different bills each month, and each possibly for a different amount. You may find that your billings have to be divided if a master subscriber pays part of the premium and the individual enrollee pays the balance. The computer database program can provide these specialized bills for you instantly.

In addition to this primary billing, the computer will handle a secondary one as well. Invariably, especially with multiple individual contracts paid individually, you will have clients who do not pay, or at least pay late. The computer can sort these clients out, and send them a second bill. Payment problems are an unfortunate but inevitable fact of business.

The computer can produce mailing labels for these clients or address individual envelopes to be billed or contacted for something. That will greatly decrease your administrative work, and increase your profit. It can then decide which providers are entitled to the capitation payment for the individual members in a given month and prepare a pay voucher and eligibility list for them as well.

When you accept members in the plan, you will have to send them an acknowledgment of that acceptance and a membership card which will identify them to the provider each time they present for treatment. The card should indicate just who is eligible and which dependents have been included in the plan. You should put a quick reference code number on the card so that you can call it up on the computer rapidly when the dentist calls or some other problem arises. The filing program of a computer can produce these cards for you at the time you enter individual records. Here again administrative work can be greatly reduced by this function, and your margin of profit will increase. You can send the cards and a thank you at the same time and give your credibility another boost. Wait though, until the payments have been received. This is after all, a paid-in-advance concept.

Summary

We have come to the end of our discussion of capitation plans. From it you should have been able to ascertain some principles. Some of them are major and deal with the concept of capitation as a whole and others are minor and deal with the day-to-day operation of the plans.

You should have learned that capitation plans are closely intertwined with HMO plans and for the most part, follow their direction. From that, it should be apparent that if you are interested in offering capitation plans directly out of your office or the offices of some of your associates, you will no doubt ultimately be required to obtain a license or certificate of authority to do so. While many states still do not have any legislation commanding such compliance, it seems inevitable that soon most will. The basic principle underlying this determination is the "assumption of risk" postulate. Capitation plans shift the risk of delivering services to the providers and that shift draws with it concern on the part of those entrusted with protecting public interest for the viability of the providers. With the inevitable requirement for licensing, capitation plans become increasingly complicated. Arduous rules and regulations require discipline, perseverance, and close communication with insurance commissioners.

That said, our discussion should have indicated that in spite of complications, the guidelines for offering capitation plans have been conveniently spelled out in the HMO laws. Using those guidelines and developing relations and contracts with providers and subscribers is not all that difficult. Designing contracts and all of the documentation for prepaid plans in general becomes only a process of weaving individual threads of logic coherently together. Subsequent management of the plan, once it is operational, is only a function of simple business organization. That organization can be greatly aided by the use of a small computer and a couple of software programs.

You should have been able to deduce that capitation plans are not for everybody. Indeed, they require considerable horsepower to run successfully. They may not be realistic for the small solo practitioner, especially in a state where governmental regulation is strong. Capitation plans can, nevertheless, be offered directly out of the dental fraternity, but only by groups of providers who have banded together, or by those with larger groups with multiple facilities and expanded staff and operational capabilities. Volume and internal cost reduction are mandatory for success, and that may be impractical for the small operator.

Finally, you may have been able to infer that capitation plans can sometimes be provider-unfriendly and that may ultimately lead to dissatisfaction on the part of the consumer. Taken together, provider distrust and consumer dissatisfaction may ultimately spell major changes in both the HMO and capitation formats. Those changes have begun to manifest themselves in the form of hybrid plans derived from the developing PPO model. It is these hybrids that are most suited to the solo practitioner who desires to entice a few local groups into visiting his practice. They may even become the mainstay of those larger groups capable of capitation delivery currently, but who see that glimmer of evolution on the horizon of health care.

SECTION III

Discount PPO-Model Plans

Chapter 9 Introduction to Discount PPO-Model Plans

Until now, we have been concentrating our efforts on establishing a dental capitation plan. Anyone reading the preceding chapters should have come to the conclusion that creating and properly managing one of these monsters requires a lot of horsepower, and probably is not the option of choice for the small operator or even a small group which intends to offer dental plans directly out of the office.

Predictably, the capitation concept will be around for a while, though some people feel that it may be a doomed species when looked at realistically. The reason? It is a provider-unfriendly system. Granted, those practitioners who have received capitation premiums and have not seen (or been required to provide many services to) patients are basking in the luxury of being paid in advance. However, it appears as though they may be a minority in the overall scheme of things. Those administrators who have shared in the premiums and taken none of the risk for providing treatment may think they have reached economic bliss as well. Unfortunately there is a small, but nonetheless detectable undercurrent of rebellion swelling among the front line practitioners. It may someday gain enough strength to overthrow the kingdom.

Provider-unfriendly? Certainly. Once you have managed to understand all of the concepts we have discussed so far, you may agree that a pure capitation plan, while being effective and easy to sell to clients, is cumbersome. Yet the concept of attracting new patients by offering a reduced fee in exchange for guaranteed loyalty to a particular practice or group of practices is an extremely viable one. Enter the concept of discounting by groups, contracting directly by providers, or the preferred provider-based plan.

The PPO and the Assumption of Risk.

Before we begin our discussion of the kind of discount plan that can be best offered directly from the individual dental office or by the smaller group, let's take a look at the progenitor of this species—the PPO. The acronym PPO stands for *Preferred Provider Organization*. The American Dental Association does not particularly care for the term "preferred provider." They feel it may tend to promote one dentist over another on the basis of skill rather than economic considerations. Therefore they have elected to use the term *Contracting Dental Organization*. For our purposes we will stick to the ubiquitous PPO.

PPOs differ from HMOs in a variety of ways. Most notably, providers under the PPO system do not share directly in any of the premiums collected from patients by third parties. They deliver their services on a fee-for-service basis. That in itself is sufficient to attract many providers disillusioned with the prepaid concept.

Indemnifying insurers assume the financial risk of providing the health care needed by their clients. They agree to pay if service becomes necessary. HMOs and the providers contracted by capitation companies do the same thing in effect, but they do not pay with dollars. Instead, they agree to provide the actual services needed by their clients. HMOs may suffer a lag time between delivery of services and collection of premiums, but essentially, in both cases, money is collected in advance and services are delivered later. These companies assume the risk of caring for a group of people regardless of how large that burden becomes. This unmitigated assumption of risk is what scares insurance commissioners. Indeed, this is why we have insurance commissioners and their litany of rules and regulations. Nobody wants anyone to collect the money and then not be able to provide the services later. That interferes with basic rights and borders on criminal activity.

PPO providers assume no such risks. They only agree to accept a lesser payment for their services when treating clients of the PPO hierarchy. Their incentive for giving away a percentage of their profit is to ensure the long range success of their practice by attracting a new congregation of patients away from the ever-increasing number of practitioners. It has been proposed by some that this voluntary dilution of profit has been at least in part initiated by the providers themselves, in a conscientious effort to reduce the cost of health care to the consumer. In many cases the PPO providers actually pay a fee to the sponsoring company for that privilege, which makes it appear to be a provider-based program to an even greater extent. The postulate seems unlikely, however, in light of how financially rewarding the indemnifying/fee-for-service system has been in the past. Who would want to give that up? A more likely scenario is that conversion to the PPO model has been promoted by the insurers and the consumers. When we analyze the situation, the cost containment is coming from the providers as usual. Have insurance companies voluntarily given up any of their profits in the interest of reducing costs to the consumer? It seems a remote possibility.

More germane is the fact that so many providers have been injected into the system over the years by social pressure, and the dictates of legislative action, that simple supply-and-demand economics have opened the door for insurers to promote the concept. It has become almost a "do-or-die" proposition for the providers in light of that competition.

Is the ultimate goal to enlist all providers into the PPO system and thereby directly control the costs of health care? Some have said yes, and that has triggered monumental questions regarding PPOs and the violation of antitrust laws and the principles of price fixing. It is an irony that this same PPO concept which threatens to subjugate the freedom of the individual practitioner to control his own affairs is the same concept which could ultimately free him of that burden, and thrust those entrepreneurs willing to gamble into a position of financial superiority again.

Organizers of PPOs are telling consumers that for a fee they will arrange for a list of providers to provide treatments at reduced charges. The consumers are paying for discounts essentially just as they would by signing up for any group purchasing club like those offered by credit card companies. Optical providers have been offering similar programs for years. In addition to the discounts, some review procedures are included to assure necessity of treatment and that the treatment conforms to accepted standards of care. The latter two products offered by the PPO concept are valuable to be sure, but they are also available from most state licensing boards, as well as from any of the many provider associations currently in existence. Consumers do not have to rely on internal control procedures for that assurance. If the system fails, a bevy of capable attorneys waits patiently for providers to contradict the recommendations of these pre-existing regulatory entities so that they can run a complaint through *their* ultimate system of review and litigation. Eventually, litigation against a particular practitioner or treatment can be sufficient enough to cause either to die out. This *peer review by natural selection* is without question increasingly effective in assuring standard of care and appropriateness of services. Providers not adhering to this ultimate system will find themselves on the economic endangered species list in short order.

The good news is that some providers are finding that they can go to the same group of subscribers solicited by the insurers and tell them that they will give them the same discounts available through the PPO, but charge them far less in group membership fees. They are eliminating the middleman insurer by virtue of their ability to monitor the system for much less. They simply do not have the overhead of a large insurer. Granted the nascent movement is small, but nonetheless each egg stolen removes a clutch of genes from the posterity of the giants. In addition, providers who have banded together to steal these eggs are finding that they can offer the same standard of treatment control offered by the bigger companies, since in the end it is the provider who makes those decisions. Indeed, many state board and insurance company case reviewers are PPO providers as well.

If we have made it sound simple, that's exactly what it is. If you are a provider, even a solo practitioner on the outskirts of civilization, you can approach a group of potential patients and offer them discounted services for a promise of fidelity. If you are smart, you will be able to attach a fee to that idea and collect your daily bread, so to speak, on both ends. The remainder of the book will address this reality.

Simple Discount Plans

If you are a practitioner participating in the consumer-mandated health care cost-containment reformation, you will in some way or another discount your services. Everybody hates the word *discount*. Providers hate to even think about it. Insurance companies avoid it so that their programs do not sound like something sold in a catalog. Even patients are leery about visiting a discount dentist. So people try not to use it. They say allowance, or reduction, or deduction, but seldom discount. But discounting is exactly what you are doing when you participate. You are agreeing to accept a lesser fee in return for a promise that patients will come to your office. The discount may be hidden in the form of a table of allowances or a schedule of maximum fees charged, but unless your fees are already very low, that discount is there. The task of the participating dentist is to learn to provide services at lower fees and still profit. Accomplishing that means decreasing expenses and increasing both patient volume and practice efficiency. You can tip the scales in your favor if you can charge a yearly membership fee to a group for the privilege of benefiting from those discounts. Your reduced salary from a purely dental operation can be offset by the membership fees and bring your overall discount back up to a respectable level.

A simple membership-fee-for-discount program, coupled with cost control and increased efficiency, is significantly easier for the solo practitioner to manage and seems a much faster and more realistic track than a capitation plan.

Legality

The nice thing about discounting is that it assumes no risk. You can offer fees to a group that are below the existing norms and not take on any responsibility for that group's total dental health. For that reason, licensing of discount plans is considerably more realistic than licensing of capitation plans.

When insurance companies first began their operations in the fifties, little question existed about the need to regulate them. Agencies were established immediately to do so. When the HMO concept appeared on the scene, people scratched their heads and asked should we regulate them or not? Do they fall under the jurisdiction of the insurance commissioners or not? Are they insurance plans? Considerable controversy over the topic ensued. For a long time many HMOs remained in operation without clear legislative policies. As we have said, that is still true in some instances with regard to dental capitation plans, although the trend is towards regulation. Soon all areas will treat capitation plans like insurance and require compliance with regulatory procedures. We are back to the head-scratching stage with the PPO concept and certainly confused about simple discount plans. The trend now, however, in contrast to the capitation concept, is toward less regulation. Indeed, many states have already decided that no legislation will be required and readily allow this type of plan. They are convinced that since the assumption of risk principle is negated, discount or PPO plans do not fall under the authority of the insurance commission.

In spite of that fact, though, some resistance to the PPO concept still exists. Some claim that if you charge a membership fee, you have accepted payment in advance for something you have not delivered. While you are not at risk to deliver anything, you are required to stay in business to make the promised deliveries when necessary. If your discounts are too low, they fear that you will indeed go out of business and won't be able to deliver the services. But instead of requiring massive assurances (which parallel the capitation rules) that you will remain viable, insurance commissions in some areas merely place limitations on the amount you can discount. It is that simple. The rules for discount plans in the state of Kentucky are a good example of the principle. When you boil them down, they merely say that you cannot discount more than 25% of what the industry norm is for a particular service. That way, the assumption is that your chances of remaining in business long enough to fulfill your promise will be higher. In addition some areas require a fidelity bond, but it is small and of no consequence when compared to capitation guidelines.

By way of contrast, the state of Michigan, which has one of the most complicated capitation regulatory systems, requires only a one-page letter outlining your intentions before granting a certificate of authority.

Licensing

Concern over licensing a simple discount program offered out of your office or preferably through an intermediate company like DMI may not be necessary. But, if you are concerned, instead of preparing a massive proposal as would be required if you wanted to offer a capitation plan, just send the insurance commission a letter outlining what you are planning. They will respond with a letter authorizing your activity on the spot or provide you with a brief description of what will be required to obtain such authority. Either way, you will find it notably easier than starting a capitation plan.

An example of a letter which would result in the granting of authority to operate a discount plan in the state of Michigan might read like this:

Dental Maintenance International
2972 Elm Street
Maple, Michigan 48888

Date

Insurance Commissioner
State of Michigan
Lansing, MI 48909

Dear Mr. Commissioner:

This letter is intended to outline the activities of Dental Maintenance International, a registered Michigan corporation.

Dental Maintenance International has entered into agreements with licensed Michigan dentists to provide discounted dental services to its clients on a fee-for-service basis. Members covered under Dental Maintenance International's programs pay a nominal yearly membership fee. In return, they are entitled to percentage discounts on services delivered by our participating provider offices exclusively.

Dental Maintenance International assumes no risk for delivery of services.

It is our understanding that this type of arrangement does not require licensing by the Michigan Department of Licensing and Regulation or the Insurance Bureau. Please affirm this in writing at your earliest convenience.

Thank you for your consideration.

Sincerely,

Your name
Dental Maintenance International

As you can see it is a very simple letter. You may, of course, need to customize it to meet requirements in your state, but simplicity is the underlying principle of PPO model plans. Our letter makes reference to "discounts on services." You may decide that offering percentage discounts is not the way you want to set up your program and you may have to adjust the letter accordingly. We will discuss the idea of fee structures and discounting in greater detail later.

Letter of Authority

A letter like the one above generated a response from the insurance office in the state of Michigan similar to the one that follows:

State of Michigan
Department of Licensing and Regulation

Dental Maintenance International
2972 Elm Street
Maple, MI 48888

Dear Sirs,

This letter is in response to your correspondence regarding the activities of Dental Maintenance International. It appears from your description that DMI will provide dental services on a discounted fee-for-service basis. Since DMI will not be operating a pre-paid dental program and will not assume financial risk for delivery of services, it is our determination that this program would not qualify as an Alternative Health Care Financing and Delivery System under Section 21042 of Public Act 368 of 1978, as amended.

Please be advised that should DMI change its operations from the one described in your letter, or should prevailing laws be changed in the future, the Insurance Bureau reserves the right to re-evaluate the program.

Sincerely,

Analyst, Office of Health Insurance.

Provider-Friendly Systems

A one-page request letter and a one-page response, and DMI is qualified to offer its plan in the state of Michigan. Obviously, it may not be quite that simple in your area, but since both of these are reproductions of actual recent letters, they serve as examples of the fact that licensing PPO modeled discount plans can be vastly simpler than licensing capitation plans. That assumes, of course, that things remain the same as they are at the time of this writing. Legislation and the feelings of insurance commissions change from time to time.

This simplicity underlies the overall friendliness of this concept. As we discuss more of the points involved and compare them to the capitation concept, you will see further evidence of this. In addition you will see why some are predicting that provider-friendly systems may gradually replace some of the conventional systems operating in the health care industry.

Chapter 10 Provider Relations in a Discount PPO Plan

Making arrangements with providers under a PPO-modeled discount plan can be much easier than when making similar arrangements under the capitation concept. Obviously if you are offering the plan directly out of your office to small groups who will come to you only, you will not require any arrangements at all. You can even use your own name in your marketing and provide the services to a limited group of people. However, establishing a separate corporation just as with the capitation company would be a better idea for all of the same reasons. Sooner or later you will want to solicit the help of some of your comrades in order to handle larger groups or more diversified groups. With this type of plan you'll find resistance to be dramatically lowered.

Solicitation Letter

As with capitation, try to solicit your friends first by word of mouth. That way you will be assured that the offices you choose will be able to handle the load. If you find that you need to solicit providers in other areas, or perhaps providers that you really do not know, you will have to do it using a solicitation letter and office questionnaire. The office questionnaire can be the same one used for a capitation plan but the solicitation letter will require some modifications to ensure that your prospective providers know that you are dealing now with a plan based on fee-for-service instead of capitation.

Regardless of the method of initial contact, most providers will respond by asking you to send them something so they can read it over and make a decision. You might as well develop such a letter or information packet if you intend to sign providers other than yourself.

An example of an initial provider solicitation letter for a discount PPO-modeled plan might look like this:

DENTAL MAINTENANCE INTERNATIONAL
2972 Elm Street, Maple, Michigan 48888

Dear Doctor,

Dental Maintenance International is an authorized administrator of dental plans in the state of Michigan. We are looking for dentists to provide services to our clients in your area.

Our dental plan is a very simple one, modeled after the Contracting Dentist Organization format. It is a provider-oriented plan. If you have examined other plans, or perhaps participated in them, we are certain you will like this one! Very simply, if you elect to become one of our Dental Maintenance International dentists, you will be asked to treat our patients on a discounted fee-for-service basis. The discounts are from your usual, customary, and reasonable fees, and do not bind you to a fixed table of allowances. Discount rates have been adjusted so that the highest discounts are on those procedures that cost you the least. Therefore you can still provide the quality services you are used to providing without having to lose your shirt to do it!

Sound interesting? In addition, you will be pleased to know that you can provide services during your normal office hours. To be a DMI provider, you do not have to expand your office unless you want to. Of course, there are no claim forms, preauthorizations, or limits of any kind. You may do exactly what you and the patient determine is necessary, and operate your practice in the professional manner you are accustomed to.

This is a basic services plan. You are not responsible for specialty services as in some other plans. You are responsible only for those services which are within your level of expertise. Specialists in the plan will deal separately with each case just as you do. Treatment of TMJ, self-inflicted wounds, occupational injuries, and a host of other services are excluded from this plan to protect your interests.

If you think the plan may be for you, please fill out the enclosed card, and someone will contact you. There is, of course, no obligation, but we will be limiting the number of providers in an effort to provide sufficient patient volume for each provider, so don't hesitate. Someone in your area **will** take the plan. It might as well be you!

Sincerely,

Dental Maintenance International

Choosing Offices

You will not need to be nearly as critical about who you allow into this plan as you might be with a capitation plan. Since the providers under this type of arrangement are not obligated to assume the risk of providing all of the treatment to your clients, determining teir ability to handle the responsibility is not as critical. If they are willing to provide the services at the discount rate, you can let them try and adjust the number of available providers as time goes on. Natural selection will help with the screening at this point. Patients, who are free under this system to travel around to any provider in the plan, will base their decisions about providers on traditional values such as convenience, price, and perception of quality. If one of your providers hasn't brought his methods or his physical plant into the twentieth century, he will have the same difficulties surviving under this plan that he is no doubt experiencing in his conventional practice. People simply will not visit him. The problem with this natural selection scenario is that it will dent your credibility a bit. So, while it will be possible for you to accept a variety of practitioners into the plan, you will still want to screen them somewhat. Your aim is to have providers that reflect positively on your name. In that regard, you should be certain that the providers you choose are capable of providing most, if not all, of the treatments outlined on your fee schedule. If you offer root canals for example, your providers should be capable of at least performing the routine ones.

Try to incorporate some specialists into the plan also to increase your credibility. They too may be much more willing to join this type of plan than a capitation plan where too much uncertainty exists concerning how they will share in the premiums. If however, you offer only a basic service plan, you may find that you can do it without specialists at all.

Provider Information Packet

We mentioned earlier that providers will invariably ask that you send them something to read and fret about for a while in their own privacy. That information packet should contain a couple of items.

First of all, you should devise a descriptive letter that outlines the features of your plan and states that you are authorized by your state licensing commission and that you are capable of administering the plan.

You should point out that this is a fee-for-service plan. These are magic words. Many providers may not know the difference between capitation, HMOs, indemnifying insurers, or dental service corporations, but they will relax a bit when they hear "fee-for-service." Point out that they will not be ultimately responsible for providing all of the necessary treatment for a given group which is signing up for services to be delivered exclusively by one office. They will only be required to provide treatment to patients if and when patients show up at the office, and then they only have to offer the treatment on your discounted-fee basis. The dentists can make all practice decisions in the same manner as usual. Make it clear that under this plan they will not be responsible for specialty treatment. The dentists will only provide the services ordinarily provided. The services of the specialist are the responsibility of the patient. Further, the explanatory letter should point out how convenient it is for the providers to get in and out of the program and how convenient it will be to use.

Fees

The next item in the provider information packet should be a list of the discounts he will have to provide for your clients. Traditionally this is handled by a variety of methods. The first method is the fixed fee schedule. This method is borrowed from the capitation format. Average existing fees are computed for a given area, and then reduced by a percentage which will make it attractive to potential patients. This discount is frequently in the 20 to 25% range, with greater reductions of up to 100% on preventive and simple procedures. Each provider in the system then must charge only these fees to the patients when they present for treatment. Some PPO administrative companies then take a percentage of each of those fees when services are delivered, further diluting the amount of money the provider receives. Unquestionably, this practice is a source of considerable dissatisfaction for the providers.

Problems with Averaging

One problem with this system has to do with averaging. To establish these numbers, companies sample the fees charged by a group of dentists in a given area and produce a fee schedule that is supposed to be representative. The discounts are then made from it. No guarantee exists that a particular doctor in the system will be granting a discount at all if his fees are already lower than the average. On the contrary, doctors with high fees may end up carrying most of the burden of discounting. Further, the averages are often established using doctor's fees in one particular metropolitan area. Providers outside the area are frequently required to adhere to those fees when in reality they may have little bearing on what they actually charge.

The entire concept of a fixed fee schedule for your PPO adds credence to the argument posed by some who consider PPOs a form of price fixing. In contrast to price fixing fostered by the actual providers of services or manufacturers of products, it appears that in this case the price fixing has been initiated by the larger insurers sponsoring the program, in an effort to control fees. Nonetheless, whether by the insurer or provider, the fees are still fixed.

Table of Allowances

A table of allowances is another form of a fixed fee schedule. In this case, a maximum allowable fee is set by the sponsor, and providers are required to charge their usual fee or the allowance fee, whichever is less. The difference between a fixed fee schedule and a table of maximum allowances is small. For some providers, the maximum rate may be above what they normally charge, and therefore it makes little difference. Those whose fees are higher may find they have to discount much deeper in order to remain in the plan.

Dual Schedules

Another practice initiated by some existing plans has caused as much dissatisfaction among general providers as the practice of extracting an additional administration fee from the gross charges. This is the practice of providing dual fee schedules, one for generalists and another for specialists. Some plan administrators (nondental in some cases) have determined that a root canal done by a specialist is always superior to one done by a generalist. This may be true in some instances, but every generalist performing a particular service likes to think, that when he completes it, it will be as good as one performed by any specialist. He refers those cases in which he feels he may not be able to do equivalent work to the specialist, and wants to be paid the same for those he does himself. It is a common theme: equal pay for equal work. Certainly, as many cases exist where the work is of equal quality as cases where the work of the specialist is superior. Dual fee schedules have caused considerable resentment on the part of providers, and strained relations between administrators and providers in some plans.

Percentage Discounts

An inexpensive way DMI might combat the problem of fee schedules for its discount plan is to make it a true percentage-discount-for-service plan. Set a fixed percentage discount for a particular service and stick to it for everyone. Let's use a root canal as an example. DMI might want to offer a discount of 25% on an anterior to enrollees in the plan. Here are some of the advantages to this format:

1. It will not be necessary to establish any averages. Gathering this type of information and keeping it current can be an expensive proposition. True, services are available that provide information at reasonable costs, but sometimes the statistics can be misleading.
2. Providers outside the area of averaging will not be required to participate in a plan based on what other providers are doing. All plan providers agree to provide services on the same percentage.
3. A second fee schedule for specialists is eliminated. They must offer the same 25% discount as the generalists. This fair handling of the problem will make generalists in the system less likely to rebel.
4. Patients visiting offices in the system will be assured that they will be indeed getting something for their money. Under another fee structure system, when a patient visits the office of a provider whose fees are already below what the maximum table of allowances establishes, he will be charged that usual fee. If he visits an office where fees are higher than the allowed fee, but not higher than the 25% discount, he will not enjoy the same savings. Where is the advantage? Under a percentage discount plan, he will be guaranteed a savings wherever he chooses to go. That will give a fantastic boost to the credibility of DMI.
5. Providers may be more willing to sign up for the system if they understand it better. Many may already be used to giving discounts on some preventive services as a loss leader to attract new patients. Local newspapers and direct mail vouchers are full of discount coupons offered to new clients by dentists. Since the same rules hold true for establishing this fee schedule, where higher discounts are given on those less costly items (exams and X-rays for example), the differences may be negligible and far more acceptable to potential providers.

6. Providers may find the program more acceptable simply because they will not have to alter their standard fee-for-service schedule. They can establish their fees at whatever level they want instead of a level determined, at least by inference, by third parties. They will be able to set their fees according to the old rule of "what the market will bear," as usual. Providers who are able to get more for their services than others based on reputation or location or whatever, will still be able to get that difference, instead of having to conform to a fee regulated by other providers.

7. Finally, it is simpler, and simplicity is an underlying precept for the success of any plan. Historically, the more complicated a plan is for both the providers and the patients, the more problems it will face and the more guarded its prognosis for success.

8. Since the discounts will be from a variety of differing office fee schedules, the final price of service will vary. This will help to refute the nagging price fixing argument.

If you are a practitioner establishing a system like this, analyze your existing fees closely. You can afford to give greater discounts on some services than you can on others. Exams, fluoride, and X-rays are good examples. On other treatments take a good look at cost cutting procedures. Can you afford to take a 20% discount on a crown, if you use a less expensive lab, utilize auxiliaries for impressions and temporaries, pour your own models and double-book the patients? Usually you can. Practice efficiency is important for cost containment. Cut frills to the bone in every aspect of your practice and set your fees accordingly. At the last minute, of course, be sure to take a look around at what the competition is offering. You'll have to be competitive if you intend to sell anything to people in your area.

State Regulations

Some states have set limits on the discounts you offer. They do not want too much discrepancy between your discounted fee and the fee that is standard for the procedure. The logic is that if you discount too deeply, you might be in danger of going out of business. Be sure to check this out before you settle on a method of setting fees.

Participation Agreement Violations

A question potential providers ask most frequently when they consider joining a plan has to do with their participation with other insurers. They are afraid that they will violate their contract and jeopardize their regular business by accepting lower fees. In light of the vast numbers of new prepaid concepts appearing in almost every dental market across the country, it seems as though this will become a minor problem. As the numbers of dentists who are participating in some sort of discount program grow, it becomes increasingly unlikely that any of the companies who require participation agreements (dental service corporations) will find it cost-effective or prudent to limit their potential provider base. Many have begun their own programs, and to enforce the guidelines of the participation agreements would only cause difficulties for their prepaid programs as well. Some have seen this writing on the wall and have made changes in their agreements to reflect this new attitude.

For example, the new wording which describes participation agreements in the solicitation information distributed by one such state Delta plan makes it possible for dentists to participate in any "arm's-length" PPO-type plan, in this manner:

> The usual fee is that fee which is the lowest fee charged. Exceptions may be made for the fees charged under bonafide arm's-length prudent purchaser agreement.

It goes on to specify exceptions for seniors and people covered under governmental assistance plans and charges reduced in the interest of professional courtesy.

That points to another fine feature of simple discount plans like this, whether based on a table of allowance or on a percentage discount, and that is that they signal an overall fee reduction for services. Any insurer should be glad to endorse such a concept. Once yours is operational, you might want to consider seeking that endorsement to further your credibility. Insurers should be in the position of encouraging participation in fee-reducing ventures instead of preventing them, especially if you offer your plan as the primary plan, and grant the same fee reductions to the insurance company or dental service corporation.

An example of a discount fee-for-service fee schedule can be found in Appendix C. Remember, your discounts may vary depending upon how well you are able to streamline your operation.

Provider Contract

As with the capitation plan, when you offer a dental plan based on the discount fee-for-service concept and include other practitioners in the system as providers, it will be necessary to tie them to the plan using a contract. Basically it can be the same one used for the capitation plan, with some obvious changes.

A suitable provider contract might begin in the usual manner by defining the principles involved.

Provider Agreement

THIS AGREEMENT is entered into this _ day of __________ , 19 ___ by and between Dental Maintenance International Inc. (hereinafter referred to as "DMI"), a duly authorized corporation, licensed to do business as a for-profit corporation and __________ DDS, individually and dba _______ a sole proprietorship, a partnership, or corporation, all of whom are licensed to practice dentistry in the State of _______ , (hereinafter referred to as the "Dentist," whether one or more).

Recitals

Next come the standard recitals. The first should mention the fact that the plan will follow the membership-for-discount approach. The remaining recitals can be simplified. It will be unlikely that you will have to include one that reminds the provider that he may have to accept other arrangements in the event that you contract with other groups in other ways. To him it will all be the same. When patients present with their card, he will have to give them the discounts. If you set your discounts at bare-bone levels in the first place, it will be unlikely that you will be able to lower them any more and still have a viable program. Flexibility when dealing with potential clients comes from the membership fee and the ways that you collect it, and that will not affect the provider.

Witnesseth:

WHEREAS, DMI is a licensed corporation providing various individuals, groups, and associations with dental care for their members under the membership/discount allowance approach; and

WHEREAS, the Dentist represents and warrants that he/she is duly licensed to provide dental services and are certified by the board of examiners, and that the Dentist desires to provide services for DMI under the terms defined herein; and

WHEREAS, DMI wishes to contract with said Dentist to provide services to members of groups and associations with whom it has agreements;

NOW, THEREFORE, the parties do mutually covenant and agree as follows:

General Provisions

It is not necessary to include a lengthy section on definitions with a simple discount provider contract as it might be with a capitation contract. The general provisions section will provide sufficient outline to cover most controversies when they arise.

The first general provision should be a clear synopsis of the intent of the plan.

General Provisions.
The following provisions are agreed to:

1. Attachment "A," "Allowance Schedule," sets forth allowances the Dentist will grant to any DMI member presenting with a valid DMI identification card.
2. Allowances are to be granted from Dentist's usual, customary, and reasonable fee schedule.
3. The Dentist agrees to provide DMI with the schedule mentioned in Section Two (2) of the general provisions of this agreement, and warrants that this is a true copy of the fees he charges his regular patients of record. Further, the Dentist agrees to provide DMI with a copy of said fees each and every time he changes them in any way, within ten (10) days of such a change.

Provision number three is necessary to resolve disputes and to protect both the provider and the administration entity. Patients may question whether they indeed have received a discount, and the updated copy of fees should be retained as proof. Provision number four obligates the provider to render service to each patient who presents to his office. This might be a good time to add a phrase that would serve the purpose of allowing additional flexibility later if you are still uncomfortable with the potential for future contract variations.

4. The Dentist agrees to render all dental services set forth in the allowance schedule to each eligible DMI member who may present to his office to the best of his ability.

   It is further understood that DMI may enter into contacts with new individuals, groups, or organizations during the term of this contract and that the Dentist shall be responsible for the delivery of services as provided herein, to those new groups as well.

It would be wise to include a provision that outlines how the provider will prioritize appointments. Inclusion of a similar provision in the subscriber contract will help to unify the treatment regimen and avoid problems later.

5. It is agreed that the Dentist shall provide services during his normal working hours. Emergency care will be available as soon as possible and in priority to all other appointments. The Dentist agrees that his office will be covered for emergencies during vacations and other periods when the office might normally be closed. Priorities in scheduling appointments shall be as follows:

   a. Emergency care

   b. First time visits for examination and treatment

   c. Regular non-emergency dental care

   At his discretion, the Dentist may charge a cancellation charge to any member who fails to keep an appointment unless the appointment is cancelled at least twenty-four (24) hours prior to the scheduled appointment. Such charge shall be no more than $10.00.

Here are some additional provisions which will serve to clarify how the dentist will be paid for scheduled services, services which are not scheduled, and what will happen if you change things later.

6. The Dentist agrees to accept his regular fee less the allowance rate as described on the allowance schedule as payment in full for services rendered, and agrees further, not to seek additional payment for services rendered from a patient now or at any time in the future in the event this contract is cancelled for any reason. In no event shall

DMI be required to pay for any services rendered by the Dentist to any member of any DMI dental plan.

7. In the event the Dentist delivers services which are not specifically described in the allowance schedule, then the Dentist should look to the member for the applicable fees. In no event shall DMI be responsible to assist the Dentist in collecting said fees.
8. DMI may, from time to time, change the allowance schedule and will notify the Dentist accordingly.

For the provider, one of the most advantageous aspects of participation in a program such as this is that his name will be published to a group of potential patients. This is what he wants. It is the advertising and solicitation of new patients into his practice that is the bedrock of the plan. Yet, it might be a good idea to include a clause that authorizes DMI to carry out that publication just in case a dispute arises later.

9. The Dentist agrees to allow DMI to publish the Dentist's name as a participating DMI dental office to any and all individuals, groups, or organizations, with whom DMI has an agreement.

Traditional insurance carriers do not mind paying a lesser amount as part of their obligations to patients. In the interest of avoiding hassles, it would be wise to set your program up as the primary carrier and allow any other carriers to enjoy the discounts you have created. You may find that this could lead to an endorsement of your plan by those carriers at a later date, and that could mean a big boost to your credibility. Include a clause that specifies this positioning.

10. In the event any member contracting with DMI presents to the Dentist for treatment under the terms of this contract, and that member has dental coverage under any other licensed third party carrier whether obtained before or after becoming a member of the DMI plan, the Dentist agrees not to bill, charge, or seek payment from said third party carrier a fee which is greater than the Dentist's usual, customary, and reasonable fee or regular fee, less the allowance rate as described by Attachment "A" herein.

Duration and Term

The rules for duration or term of this agreement do not vary from those used for a capitation plan. You will most likely establish one-year contracts with your patient groups, so follow that guide for your provider contract as well.

> **Duration of Agreement.** This agreement shall continue until terminated by the Dentist upon ninety (90) days prior written notice to DMI or terminated by DMI upon ninety (90) days written notice to the Dentist.
>
> **Term.** This agreement shall be in effect as of the date of execution hereof and shall remain in effect for a period of one (1) year. Further, this agreement shall automatically renew each and every year hereafter, for a period of one (1) year upon the same terms and conditions.

Independent Relations and Malpractice

The next two clauses do not vary from the wording found in the capitation contract. We do not want to interfere with the way he practices and we want to specify that he maintain adequate malpractice coverage.

> **Independent Relationships.** It is specifically agreed and understood that in performing the services herein described, the Dentist is acting as an independent contractor and not as an agent or employee of DMI. The Dentist shall maintain the dentist-patient relationship with the members with whom DMI has contracted, and shall be solely responsible to the patient for the dental advice and treatment. It is expressly agreed that neither the individuals, groups, or organizations contracted with, nor DMI shall have dominion or control or the Dentist's practice or procedures, or the Dentist's personnel or facilities. The Dentist hereby agrees to hold harmless, defend, and indemnify DMI and any of its contracting groups and organizations, its board of directors, officers, employees, agents, or administrators from any claims, suits, demands, actions, etc., that may arise out of any alleged malpractice or negligent act or omission to act, caused or alleged to have been caused by the Dentist or any of his agents, employees, consultants, associates, owners, or partners in the performance or omission of any professional duty assumed by the Dentist hereunder.

Malpractice Insurance. The Dentist shall, at all times, maintain adequate malpractice insurance with a recognized insurance carrier, and shall upon demand supply DMI with a copy of said policy.

Should DMI be forced to defend itself in any lawsuit, claim, demand, or action for any malpractice or negligence on the part of the Dentist, the Dentist agrees to pay any liabilities, attorney's fees, court costs, or other expenses associated with said defense.

Eligibility

The next provision explains that DMI will handle the determination of eligibility and will serve to remind the dentist of how the plan works.

Eligibility. DMI, in conjunction with any groups or organizations with whom it has contracted, shall make all determinations of eligibility for benefits of any person under this contract. Only patients presenting to the Dentist with valid DMI identification cards shall be eligible for services under the terms of this contract. If a patient presents for treatment and does not have a valid eligibility card, the Dentist may contact DMI by telephone to ascertain whether said member is eligible before refusing to provide services under this agreement.

Exclusions and Limitations

It is not necessary to add provisions that specify office hours or waiting times for appointments under a discount PPO-modeled plan. It is basically fee-for-service as usual. When screening your potential providers, make certain that their hours and methods of scheduling are acceptable and then you can eliminate those governing clauses from your contract. You won't need to spend time worrying about the specialty problem with your discount plan either. The dentist simply isn't responsible. His only obligation is to provide the services he routinely provides on a discount basis. Try to incorporate specialists into your program to help with your credibility, but make the patients understand in their contract that specialty services are their responsibility. This simplicity is clearly an advantage over capitation. Your discount provider contract can move directly into any exclusions and limitations you may want to include. Listed below are some that are appropriate.

Exclusions and Limitations. The Dentist shall not be responsible for:

1. Any dental service not specifically described in the Allowance Schedule.
2. Any new service or procedure after the last day of the month during which any member ceased to be eligible for coverage under the group's plan with DMI. However, procedures in progress shall be completed. These procedureswill include dental treatment where an impression has been taken and/or procedures on any tooth upon which treatment has been started.
3. Visits to or services performed by a specialist, dentist, or professional not participating with DMI.
4. Any dental services arising out of any sickness or injury arising out of or sustained in the course of any occupation or employment for remuneration or profit, where member may be eligible for workman's compensation benefits, or any reimbursement through any public program, state or federal, or any program of medical or dental benefits sponsored and paid for by the federal government or any agency thereof.
5. Any dental services which, in the judgment of the Dentist are not necessary and reasonable for the prevention, correction, or im- provement of a condition.
6. Any dental services necessitated as a result of a condition sustained in the commission of a felony.
7. Oral surgery requiring the setting of fractures or dislocations.
8. Treatment of cysts or neoplasms.
9. Dispensing of drugs for treatment of oral disease not normally supplied in a dental office.
10. Prescription drugs.
11. Congenital defects.
12. Conditions affecting the temporomandibular joint including dysfunction and/or malfunction.
13. Any costs or expenses incurred in the event the participant is hospitalized for any dental procedure.
14. Services of an anesthetist or anesthesiologist.
15. Any dental charges incurred for the treatment of obesity.

16. Appliances necessary to increase vertical dimension or to restore an occlusion.
17. Programs or treatments which were in progress prior to the date any person became a participant under this plan.
18. Dental services provided at home or any nursing or rest home.
19. Special requests by patients for customized techniques differing from standard procedures will be provided at additional fees determined by the Dentist. Patients must bear the difference between the plan fees and the special fees.
20. Treatment of patients who in the judgment of the Dentist are untreatable children, or emotionally disturbed adults.
21. This plan specifically excludes any treatments that are of such complexity that they cannot be performed by the Dentists under contract with DMI.

Miscellaneous Clauses

One necessary function of the contract is to specify how the dentist will treat work in progress. We do not want any disputes arising from things left undone in the patient's mind. This will hurt not only the credibility of DMI but that of the dentist as well.

Work in Progress. In the event of termination of this contract, or termination of the contract between DMI and the group, or loss of eligibility of the member, the Dentist shall be responsible for completing work started prior to the termination of said contract or contracts, as follows:

1. If an impression has been taken the Dentist shall complete a denture or partial.
2. Work on each individual tooth which may have been started shall be completed.

The remainder of the provisions are standard and self- explanatory.

Effects of Legislation. In the event that legislation or regulations are passed or imposed by any duly constituted authority which affect the terms and conditions of this agreement, or the prepaid dental plans offered by DMI, then the parties to this agreement shall promptly attempt to comply with the provisions of such legislation by amending and revising this agreement. In the event compliance with such legislation or regulations is attempted, but the parties to this agreement are unable to accomplish such compliance within a reasonable time, then this agreement shall terminate without further obligation of either of the parties to the other.

Standard of Care. The Dentist shall in no way differentiate in the quality of treatment, days of treatment, or time of day of treatment, between DMI patients and his own private patients.

Inclusion of the Dentist on the panel of providers is not necessarily a recommendation of said Dentist by DMI.

Nonexclusivity. This contract is mutually nonexclusive. DMI, participating groups or organizations, or individual members of such groups are entitled to enter into similar contracts with other dentists. The Dentist is also free to enter into other contracts with other prepaid companies, other groups, and any others not represented by DMI, and to maintain his private practice as well.

Advertising. In the event the Dentist advertises in any manner whatsoever, the Dentist shall not use DMI's name without first and on each occasion obtaining written consent from DMI.

Confidential Information. The Dentist acknowledges that DMI has invested substantial time, expertise and expenses in creating prepaid dental plan documentation. The Dentist agrees that this documentation is the property of DMI and will be kept confidential and used by the Dentist only for the purposes for which it is devised.

Modification and Assignability. This agreement contains the entire and complete understanding between the parties.

Because of the nature of the services to be performed, this agreement shall not be assignable by the Dentist, nor shall the benefits thereof be passed on to and naturalized by the Dentist's heirs and/or successors in interest. DMI shall be entitled to assign this agreement to its heirs, representatives, successors, and/or assigns without limitation.

Dental Records. All dental records, including billing information, for members of groups contracting with DMI shall be retained by the Dentist for a period of at least five (5) years after the date of said member's last visit to the office. DMI and/or its agents or representatives shall be entitled to inspect said records upon reasonable written request.

Notices. Whenever it becomes necessary for either party to serve notice on the other respecting the terms of this contract, such notice shall be served by certified mail, return receipt requested, addressed as indicated below:

(a) Dental Maintenance International
123 Elm Street
Maple, MI 48888

(b) John Q. Dentist
Somewhere Street
Somewhere, U.S.A.

Closing

The contract closes in the usual manner.

IN WITNESS WHEREOF, the parties have caused this agreement to be executed as of the date mentioned on page one.

Dentist	**DMI**
by: ______________________	**by:** ______________________

Dental Maintenance International

Address __________________	Address __________________
City _____________________	City _____________________
State/ZIP ________________	State/ZIP ________________
Phone ___________________	Phone ___________________

Administrative Charges

The only other clause you might want to include in your contract is one dealing with the administrative cut some companies take from the gross billings of the dentist. A common way this is handled is to insert a clause that specifies that the dentist will not bill the insurance carriers directly but will send any billings directly to the PPO administration company, which will then forward them to the insurer for payment. When the money is received, the company takes its cut (usually 10%), and mails the balance to the dentist. This practice is very unpopular with the providers. They have already done their part toward cost containment and are angered when a third party takes a slice of the health care dollar in the form of a membership fee and then another slice in the form of a percentage of gross billings. That last slice is too much, since it further reduces the overall payment the dentist receives. Some PPO administration companies have reacted to this problem by dropping this charge and have resolved themselves to accepting only the membership fee as compensation for establishing the PPO network and putting the doctors and the patients together. Who knows what the future will bring? If you want to grab another slice of the pie for your efforts, then include such a clause. It might read like this:

> The Dentist shall submit to DMI all billings for health care services provided to any patient under contract to DMI for dental services.
>
> The Dentist agrees to pay DMI an administrative fee of ten (10%) percent of the gross billings from the maximum fee schedule charged to patients or any other third party carrier contracting with DMI.

Patient Encounter Forms

Record keeping is considerably more complicated for the capitation plan than it is for the simple discount plan we have just described. It is a necessary function, however, and one mandated by regulation. If dentists are to be paid based on the amount of work they do using a dental service unit approach and the risk pool concept, it is very important. Simplification is one of the attractive features of the discount plan. Technically, in that interest, the patient encounter form, so necessary in the capitation format, can be eliminated all together when using the discount PPO plan. The administration company does not really care how many times a patient visits one of its providers or how much treatment is delivered. It doesn't matter. Simplification is the big advantage of this idea.

Some might disagree because having some utilization statistics can be valuable when contract negotiation time rolls around. It can be helpful to point out to prospective new clients, or to old ones who are wondering whether to renew or not, just how valuable the plan has been. Dazzling them with some statistics about how much they have saved collectively can be a sales aid. But, if your plan truly has been successful, they will already know that. If they don't wish to re-sign because they perceive that their work has been completed, no statistics in the world will help you to change their minds.

There might be some value to having an encounter form to help determine the appropriateness of treatment. But here again, the administration company does not really care that much. If a patient and a doctor agree that a particular treatment is appropriate, then it is.

Nonetheless, if you feel that you would like to encumber your plan with an encounter procedure, use the form outlined in the capitation section.

Chapter 11 Subscriber Relations

Managing potential clients when using a discount PPO-modeled plan is, in many ways, similar to managing them under a capitation format. But the discount plan format is so uncomplicated, in comparison, that you will find many of the problems intrinsic to capitation simply nonexistent.

Membership Fees

Prospective clients will have the same question when you approach them with this idea that they would have with capitation or any other plan. They will want to know what they will get and how much they will have to pay. They will be considerably less interested in all of the technical aspects of the plan such as the method in which the dentists are paid, or utilization complexities. Your task is to simply answer that first question.

We discussed the establishment of co-pay fees in the preceding chapter. If you have done it correctly and are offering the plan directly out of your office, you can set your membership fee at a rate that will net almost what you would have on a strict fee-for-service basis. Your dual roles as dentist and director of the prepaid administration company will allow you to receive two salaries, which when added together, should generate a respectable result. Make sure though, the membership fee for a given family, and the co-pays (for routine preventive services with no other work) add up to less than they would have spent on a purely fee-for-service basis. In other words, subscribers must save money right up front, or the plan will be difficult to sell.

The capitation fee principles of community rating and experience rating do not apply to this system. In fact you can sell this program to single individuals or groups at different rates with total impunity. Set the fee so that the single individual as well as families will save money. Then, drop the rate on a graduated basis, depending on the size of the group. Obviously, your administrative effort both in terms of marketing and management will be proportionately less with larger groups, so lowering the fee will not affect your expenses. The greater lump-sum membership fee from a larger group is a very attractive compensation and making the membership fee smaller to those larger groups is a valuable marketing tool.

An example of a graduated member/group fee schedule for the PPO-modeled discount plan can be found in Appendix D. The example is based on the fees for one office in the Midwest. You may find that the numbers will be different for your area, as will the rates when compared to the competition. In this schedule, advantages are cumulative. That is, an individual who signs up for the plan, but is not a member of a group, will save money on a yearly basis for routine prevention. Obviously he will save even more if he requires any work. That savings will increase if he takes a child or a spouse into the plan and will continue to increase incrementally as the number of members of his family grows. Savings increase in basically the same manner for those individuals belonging to a group. As the group size increases, so do the savings.

Are you giving up too much? Ask yourself how much you would be willing to spend to attract a cluster of patients the size of one of the groups mentioned in the schedule. What would you spend on conventional marketing for a group that large? Keep the benefits in mind. One happy customer has a direct influence on at least five other customers. Take whatever you can. Your competition is.

A final word about membership fees. Take a look around at the competition before you settle on the amounts. Remember, you are competing with other companies because of your increased efficiency and reduced overhead. Make sure your fees reflect that. If you cannot offer a plan that dramatically differs in fees from conventional plans, you will not find it very marketable.

Choosing Client Groups

You can market your discount plan to any of the same basic groups as you could with capitation: individuals, employer/employee groups, and associations. The difference is it is easier than marketing a capitation plan. This type of plan is perfect for the individual or single family. If you design your membership rate schedule on a sliding scale based on numbers of members, as we have suggested, the individual will be on the top of the list. That is, the individual will have to pay the highest rate. True, their utilization will probably be high but that is of no consequence to us under this system. More importantly, the sliding scale offers an incentive for more people to sign up from a given potential group and thereby increase overall revenues. But, since they pay the fee one time at the beginning of the period, we are not concerned with the problems of continuous monthly billings, or with an employer who has to send in a check each month from payroll deductions. That provides a wider latitude for screening potential groups.

The discount PPO-modeled plan is essentially an individual plan in all of its aspects. This makes it perfect for the association or club which may not have any financial control over its members. Instead of trying to contract with the master group and then trying to figure out a method for them to pay for the members who sign up, you can settle for a number of individual arrangements linked by a common fee based on numbers. You will not have to contract with the master group at all, and this will simplify your marketing effort dramatically.

The collection of the total premium in advance is truly a "prepaid" concept. If you have not received the premium, you do not issue membership cards and consequently patients are not entitled to treatment. This makes relations with employer/employee groups easier as well. Instead of trying to talk an employer into taking the responsibility for collecting the fees of his employees, and ultimately for the financial impact of that fee sometime in the future, you will only have to convince him to collect it one time, or at least allow you access to his employees for direct marketing with no participation from him at all. That is an idea you will find considerably easier to sell.

The only major principle to adhere to is to make sure your fee schedule is significantly slanted so that it is obvious that participation by larger groups is financially advantageous. That will help with sales too.

One last point about choosing groups for a plan like this: A typical PPO—one started by an insurance company or a dental service corporation or a separate company that has forced its way in between the insurer and the dentist—usually administers the plan for existing clients. When they create a plan for existing clients, all they are doing is asking the provider to accept less for his services. If they already have a plan, patients will have already chosen a dentist and as most providers know, will opt to stay with that plan so that they can visit him. It is only a small percentage of patients who have an existing plan and opt to switch to another plan and another practitioner just because of the money. If a practitioner becomes a provider under such a plan, those same patients will gladly switch to the new plan and stay with the doctor. Clearly then all the doctor has done is to reduce his fee for those existing patients. That only benefits the insurance company and the patients. Since the dentist does not receive any new patients out of the deal, he really does not benefit at all.

If an insurer-based PPO offers the plan to the large group, let them. Unless you have a lot of horsepower, you will find it difficult to compete.

Think of this type of plan as one which you will offer to everybody else. All the smaller fish added together will form a substantial group. This plan is best suited for those who have no other options. Our original motto of staying small at first and building slowly applies here too. But that is not to say that you should not take anything that comes along. It only means that you will find it easier at first to stick with this smaller market until you grow.

Your Own Patients

There is, however, a down side to this scenario. The primary reason for developing a capitation plan or a discount PPO-modeled plan out of your office is to attract new patients. It is certain that in the process you will have to offer the plan to patients who already visit your office. That means that you will end up only giving a discount to your existing clients. This is one of the major deterrents that keeps some practitioners from becoming providers. Don't think in terms of what you will loose, but rather concentrate on what you will gain. The next time a patient rejects your offer to build that nice three-unit bridge because they simply did not have the thousand or so dollars you ask for, why not offer them a way to reduce that fee and go ahead with the treatment? If you are administering the plan directly out of your office, you will be receiving the membership fee through your alternate identity as the prepaid company, and that will offset some of your perceived loss. In addition, you will have gained at least some of the profit from the bridge, and that in comparison to the big zero you would have received if you accepted the patient's rejection, is compensation. In another scenario, aren't there families in your practice who come in only every two to three years because of financial considerations, when in reality they should be having at least preventive services every six months or so? If you collect the membership fee from them, you will have collected more than you would have if they didn't come in at all.

On the side, when you sign a patient to a plan like this, you have welded their loyalty to your practice. You will not have to worry that when you don't see them for a long time they are visiting one of your competitors. Indeed, if they are loyal to your practice for financial reasons, it is your competitors who should worry that you will attract more of them for the same reasons. The point is that it is better to offer the plan to your existing patients who become aware of it and accept the discounted fees rather than get nothing at all.

Solicitation Letter

Once you have targeted the groups you intend to approach with your plan, you will need a method to facilitate that approach. Obviously the rules about word of mouth hold true. Try to find an opportunity to speak directly with a leader of the group and try to convince him to sign his friends or coworkers into the plan.

If you have no leads or have already signed as many patients as possible by word of mouth, you will have to use a more generalized approach. Radio, television, and newspaper advertising can be helpful in this regard, but one of the most effective and least costly means is the use of a general solicitation letter.

You may find that you will have to develop more than one: one that you send to individuals, one for clubs or associations, and another aimed at businesses in your area. Each letter should contain elements that are specifically attractive to that particular group. Your letter to individuals might stress the practitioners involved and the overall cost effectiveness of the plan. The letter to the associations might stress the fact that this plan is one of the few that can be offered to associations at all. You might have it point out that it has been sanctioned by a central managing body like the association's national office. If you are sending it to a small business in your area, you might want to stress the plan's flexibility and the fact that the employer does not really have to contribute to the plan if he does not want to.

Since it is likely that these small businesses will be one of your first targets for this discount plan, the following will serve as an example of a general business solicitation letter.

Dental Maintenance International
123 Elm Street
Maple, Michigan 48888

Dear Friends,

Good news! Dental Maintenance International is now offering selected businesses in your county an opportunity to participate in a program that could, **without cost,** add a dental plan to existing employee benefit packages. That's right. Now you can provide dental coverage for your employees at absolutely no cost to you. Of course, if you would like to contribute to the plan, that option is always open, and flexible, so that you can determine exactly how you will use it.

Sound interesting? Dental Maintenance International has been administering small dental plans in this area for several years (months). With the help of selected county dentists, these plans have been very successful. Recently, we have redesigned the program to conform to changing requirements imposed by the insurance office. This redesign has assured that our programs meet current legal standards, and has made it possible for us to incorporate other dental facilities across the county into the system.

Our programs are strictly voluntary. Only those employees who wish to participate are invited to join. There are no minimum subscriber numbers before the plan is operational. This helps to assure that people who do not need services do not end up paying for those who do!

To outline the plan briefly: Participants pay a small yearly membership fee, which then entitles them to substantial discounts every time they visit a Dental Maintenance International dental office. It couldn't be simpler! Membership rates vary depending on the size of the group, but we are certain your employees will find them attractive at any level.

Let me repeat: Your financial participation is not necessary!

I would like the opportunity to meet with you and answer any questions you may have and to explain the program to you in greater detail. If you are interested, please contact me at 555-4323.

Kindest regards,

Your name
Dental Maintenance International

After the Sale

If your initial solicitation letter is effective, or you have received inquiries from an employer, for example, who has seen some of your other advertising methods, you will have to prepare an information packet that clearly outlines the plan. You will have to meet with your prospective client or at least send this information packet to him. You will have to demonstrate your ability to handle each aspect of administering the plan for him. You will have to obtain his consent to do that administration.

Letter to Members

The first task you will have to assume if the employer agrees to endorse your plan is to notify his employees that your plan is available. Obviously, you should try to get the employer to help you in this regard, either through direct word of mouth approaches to his employees, through a newsletter if one exists (they often do with larger associations), through a note or letter in their pay envelopes, or some other method. Some employers may be willing to handle all of this function; some may be willing to handle none of it. In any event, you will have to develop a method for letting the individual members of a group know that they can now take advantage of your discount plan. You may want to use a letter like the one suggested below. You may want to send it to the members and then follow up with an information packet to those members who express an interest, or you may want to send an information packet to each member on the assumption that most of them are going to sign up.

Dental Maintenance International

Dear Friend,

Good News! Your employer has entered into an agreement with Dental Maintenance International to provide you with a comprehensive dental plan, that can save you dollars when you need a dentist.

Dental Maintenance International has developed a valuable discount dental plan for small groups exactly like yours. We are fully authorized to offer our plan to you by the Insurance Division of the State Board of Licensing. It is a basic service plan intended to help small groups and those considered "uncoverable" by conventional insurance companies to take a bite out of the high cost of dental services. Groups who have taken advantage of this opportunity have found it a very effective method of cutting costs while maintaining a simplicity unique in the industry.

You will find an information packet and an application enclosed with this letter. It should answer many of your questions, but if you still need help, please feel free to call our office at 555-4323, or contact someone at our headquarters dental office in __________, at 555-3779.

Dental Maintenance International has a rapidly expanding program. We are adding more doctors to the plan as fast as we are adding more groups. Under this system, you are not limited to a particular doctor.

You may visit any participating Dental Maintenance International provider as many times as you want. Your treatments are not limited either. The doctors in our system are free to offer you the best in time-tested, quality dental services without the restrictions imposed by other systems. We will keep you informed of increases in our provider base periodically.

With this plan, even those who do not belong to large unions or auto companies can finally benefit from dental services at prices far below industry norms. If you wish to join our family of cost-conscious people, please fill out the application at the back of the information packet, enclose a check to Dental Maintenance International for the yearly premium, and mail it to us at the address above. When we receive it, we will mail your member cards to you, and you may begin receiving treatment from one of our providers immediately.

Thank you again for your interest. We are looking forward to helping you save dollars on quality health care.

Sincerely,

Your name
Dental Maintenance International

You may find it necessary to alter this letter in a couple of ways. If you decide not to send a complete information packet to each member of the group because of the cost, or you perceive that it may be an exercise in futility, then you may want to explain in your letter that information packets are available at the personnel office or the association headquarters. If the employer has agreed to contribute to the plan or at least to help out by collecting membership fees by way of a payroll deduction, then you will have to change the letter to reflect those circumstances.

Information Packet

The information packet serves two purposes. First of all, it explains the entire plan to individual members so that their questions will be answered up front. Therefore, it will act as a master guide for the plan to be referred to in the event of a dispute. Secondly, it will act as a contract of sorts to bind the members to the plan without the formality of a standard contract. That is one of the beauties of this type of arrangement and a big surprise to many practitioners who want to set this type of concept in motion. You really do not need a specialized contract to make it work. Indeed, some practitioners have accomplished the goal of signing patients into a discount plan and collected premiums for it by using only a simple explanatory brochure. Be sure to check with your attorney to make certain that the wording is appropriate for your state, but if you follow the basic outline below, you shouldn't have any difficulties. Be sure to highlight the important aspects in your informational section and then refer back to that section on your application just before the signatures, and you will have the basis for an agreement which should be satisfactory for the amount of money and risk involved.

Dental Maintenance International
Group Dental Plan Application Packet

INTRODUCTION

The Dental Maintenance International (DMI) dental program is an affordable dental plan designed for people who are not covered by any other type of dental insurance. Participating members pay a yearly DMI membership fee. DMI contracts with dentists to provide services to eligible members at special allowance rates. There are:

- **NO TROUBLESOME CLAIM FORMS**
- **NO YEARLY MAXIMUMS**
- **NO PREAUTHORIZATIONS REQUIRED**
- **NO LIMITS**

Membership in the dental plan will entitle you to valuable allowances on all dental services delivered at the Dental Maintenance International Headquarters office in __________ and at any additional Dental Maintenance International dental offices in your area. If you compare the high cost of dental services in today's changing health care market, we are certain you will agree that this plan can save you money. For example, a family of four signing up for the plan as part of a group of 10–20 other subscribers could save $ _____ or more if all they ever need is routine maintenance. If just one member of the family should require a root canal post and crown (a common dental treatment with today's technology), you could save as much as $ __________ or more, and if you are one who anticipates the need for extensive dental treatment, your savings could be very significant. In addition, the Dental Maintenance Plan covers cosmetic dentistry. That is something most other plans exclude.

HOW DO I SIGN UP?

The rules and regulations of this plan are specified below. Read them carefully, so that you will have a full understanding of how the plan works, and then if you would like to apply for membership in the plan, fill out the application on the last page of this information package, and mail it to Dental Maintenance International at the address above.

HOW MUCH WILL I HAVE TO PAY?

When you are accepted in the plan, Dental Maintenance International will send you a bill for the first year's membership (based on the number of members who sign up) and your acceptance notification. A member allowance rate schedule for various services is enclosed with this application. In addition, a fee schedule from the   office is included so that you can see just how much money you can save by belonging to the dental plan. Fees at other offices in the system may vary, and this schedule should be used for informational purposes only. Allowance rates, however, are valid at any Dental Maintenance International Dental Office.

Remember! Those of you whose employers have agreed to pay your membership fee through payroll deductions must sign the "payroll deduction" portion at the bottom of the application.

WHEN CAN I START RECEIVING TREATMENT?

When we receive your check, we will send you a validation card, which you can present at the dental office to receive your allowances and, since there are no claim forms or authorizations necessary, you can start saving money on dental treatments immediately.

RULES AND REGULATIONS

1. All Dental Maintenance International dental plans are strictly voluntary. You do not have to sign up if you do not want to. However, if you are a member of a group, you must sign up during your group

sign-up period to qualified for group allowance rates. There is only one group sign-up period each year.

2. Services are available at the allowance rates at the _______ Dental Center and participating Dental Maintenance Plan offices only.
3. Allowances are from the usual, customary, and reasonable fee schedules of the individual offices in the program, therefore actual dollar amounts might differ depending upon which office you visit. The fee schedule included in this package is for the _______ office only!
4. This is a basic services plan. Only those services specifically mentioned in the allowance schedule are available at the allowance rate. Should members require unusual treatments not covered on the allowance schedule, the plan will not be in effect. If you require services from specialists not currently participating in the plan, the allowances will not be in effect.
5. Preventive visits which include initial oral exams, recall oral exams, routine diagnostic X-rays, routine cleaning, and fluoride treatments are limited to two a year under the plan.
6. Members are not required to sign up for a particular office. They may visit any participating office any time they wish.
7. Allowance rates mentioned in the allowance schedule are for the class of treatment involved, not just for the specific service mentioned. For example, the schedule mentions an allowance for a "two surface silver filling." Single surface and triple surface fillings are covered at the same allowance rate. The schedule also mentions "upper or lower partial." In this case the allowance rate applies to variations of a partial which may be designed at the discretion of the participating dentist.
8. Procedures performed strictly for cosmetics include bonding, laminate composite veneers, and laminate porcelain veneers.
9. Membership is in effect for one year only, beginning the day the membership fee is received by Dental Maintenance International. Procedures specifically in progress at the time membership expires will be completed at the allowance rate. Further allowances on services will not be allowed until the renewed membership fee is received by Dental Maintenance International.

10. "Primary subscriber" means the employee of an employer group, member of an association, union, or other organization who is deemed eligible for coverage under the plan by Dental Maintenance International.

11. "Eligible Dependent" means the lawful husband or wife of a primary subscriber (herein called the spouse) if no judicial decree of separation has been obtained, and such of the unmarried children of the participant from birth to the age of nineteen (19), or such of the unmarried children as are between the ages of nineteen (19) to twenty-three (23), and who are classified as full-time students at an accredited educational institution. For purposes of the preceding sentence, the term "educational institution" shall mean only an educational institution which normally maintains a regular faculty and curriculum and normally has a regularly organized body of students in attendance at the place where its educational activities are carried on.

12. "Families" mean the primary subscriber and any eligible dependents meeting the requirements of paragraph eleven (11) above, as designated by the primary subscriber.

13. APPOINTMENTS. It is agreed that participating DMI dentists shall be obligated to render services during their normal working hours only. Additional hours shall be available at the discretion of the dentist. Priorities for scheduling appointments shall be as follows:

    a. Emergency care

    b. First time visits for examination and treatment

    c. Regular non-emergency dental care

Any participant (including a dependent) who fails to keep an appointment shall be subject to a charge by the participating Dental Maintenance International dental office, unless the appointment is cancelled at least twenty-four (24) hours prior to the scheduled appointment and such charge shall be no more than $10.00.

14. EFFECT ON WORKER'S COMPENSATION. This Plan does not fulfill any requirement of worker's compensation or other compulsory insurance and cannot be used in lieu thereof.

15. THIRD PARTY RIGHTS LIMITED. All rights and liabilities created under this plan shall be deemed to exist only as between Dental Maintenance International and the primary subscriber and any

eligible dependents signing this agreement. In no event shall this plan or agreement be deemed to confer any right on or create any obligation to any third party not a signatory to the agreement or to create in such third party a status of third party beneficiary.

16. TRANSFERABILITY. This plan is expressly nontransferable.

17. FUNCTION OF Dental Maintenance International. On behalf of the primary subscriber, and his eligible dependents, DMI has arranged for the services of qualified, licensed professionals and their staffs to participate in the plan herein described. The members shall be entitled to those allowances described in the Allowance Schedule, a copy of which is attached hereto and incorporated by this reference.

DMI shall not (and does not agree nor shall it be required to) perform any dental services or do anything herein (notwithstanding any provisions hereof) that would, under applicable laws and regulations, constitute the practice of dentistry. Any provision of this agreement to the contrary notwithstanding, the sole responsibility and obligation of DMI shall be to engage in the design and administration of this plan and to use its best efforts to obtain the services of qualified, licensed professionals and their staffs to provide and perform the applicable available dental services to eligible participants. It is expressly agreed that under no circumstances shall DMI ensure that the services of such licensed professionals and their staffs will be available at any time or that the services described in the Allowance Schedule will be performed at any time. Further, under no circumstances will DMI be required to indemnify or hold harmless the Primary Subscriber, Eligible Dependent, or any Member from any cost or expense incurred in procuring any "Available Dental Services" as defined herein. All participants shall be entitled to the allowance benefits, but only to the extent that DMI shall have succeeded in obtaining the services of qualified professionals and their staffs to provide the same. The professional services will be provided and available only by the dental offices designated by DMI.

18. Dental Maintenance International reserves the right to refuse membership to individuals at its discretion.

EXCLUSIONS AND LIMITATIONS

This plan does not include the following:

1. Visits to or services performed by a specialist, dentist, or professional not participating in the plan

2. Any dental services arising out of any sickness or injury arising out of or sustained in the course of any occupation or employment for remuneration or profit, which qualifies for workmen's compensation benefits
3. Any dental services which, in the judgment of the dentist, are not reasonable and necessary for the prevention, correction, or improve ment of a condition
4. Any dental services not specifically described in the Allowance Schedule (including hospital charges or prescription drug charges)
5. Any dental services which are necessitated as a result of a self-inflicted condition
6. Any dental services for which the participant is reimbursed, entitled to reimbursement, or is in any way indemnified for such expenses by or through any public program, state or federal, or any program of medical or dental benefits sponsored and paid for by the federal government or any agency thereof
7. Any dental services necessitated as a result of a condition sustained in the commission of or the attempt to commit a felony
8. Oral surgery requiring the setting of fractures or dislocations
9. Treatment of malignancies, cysts, or neoplasms
10. Dispensing of drugs for treatment of oral disease which are not normally supplied in a dental office
11. Congenital defects
12. Conditions affecting the temporomandibular joint including dysfunction and/or malocclusion
13. Any costs or expenses incurred in the event the participant is hospitalized for any dental procedure
14. Services of an anesthetist or anesthesiologist
15. Any dental charges incurred for treatment of obesity
16. Appliances or restoration necessary to increase vertical dimension or to restore an occlusion
17. Programs or treatment which were in progress prior to the date any person became a member of this plan

18. Any new services or procedures performed after the last day during which any person ceased to be eligible for participation in this plan

19. Services which are of such complexity that they cannot be performed by the designated Dental Maintenance Plan dentists participating in the plan

As you can see, these rules and regulations are adapted directly from contracts we have used before in both the capitation plans and both of the provider contracts. The old concept of weaving the threads of federal legislation for HMOs back through all of our documentation has not changed.

The rules and regulations also outline the method we will use to administer the plan, establish membership rates and collect the premiums. If you have elected to use a sliding membership rate schedule that varies depending on the number of members, as we have suggested, you will not really know how much to charge without knowing how many people will sign up. All you can do is to provide a list of all of the membership fees (Appendix D) and then bill them later, once you know. Since they cannot receive treatment without presenting a valid membership card, and you will not issue the cards until you have received their check, you are covered financially. This is truly a paid-in-advance concept and is far superior to any monthly premium you might receive under capitation. You expect 100% utilization and are paid for it!

If you do not want to wait or cannot wait to see how many will sign up and then bill accordingly, then you will have to guess at the membership rate. You can make it the same as the number of potential subscribers if you want, but you will usually come out on the short end of the stick since the number of people who actually sign up is usually considerably lower than the number of potential subscribers. That's worth repeating. Keep in mind that the number of actual subscribers will always be lower than you expected. Even the largest insurers have learned this lesson. In the smaller companies, those just starting, or those with credibility and poor track records, it can be a source of considerable depression. Remember, you must start somewhere, and if you treat people honestly and amicably, your horsepower will grow and your company will flourish.

Application

The actual application should be the last part of your brochure, or in this case, the last part of your rules and regulations section. It should be numbered in sequence to reflect that it is part of something else. It is here that your members affix their signatures and acknowledge that they have read the rules and regulations and understand the plan completely. If your employer has agreed to use payroll deductions to collect the membership fee, be sure to include a section on your application for the members to authorize those deductions from their salaries. An example of this all-important page is shown below.

DMI Membership Application

Primary Subscriber ______________________ SOC SEC # _________

SEX M F Date of Birth __________ Phone ______________________

Address ____

City ________________________ County __________ State __________

ZIP ________ Employer or Group ______________________________

Spouse ______________________________ Date of Birth ___________

Other dependents you wish to enroll:

Child __________ Date of Birth _____ Child __________ Date of Birth

Child __________ Date of Birth _____ Child __________ Date of Birth

I/we have read the terms of the Dental Maintenance International dental program enclosed in this packet. We do hereby apply for membership in the plan. We understand the rules and regulations of the plan as defined on this application and agree to be bound by the terms and conditions of the plan as herein defined. We agree to pay Dental Maintenance International an annual membership fee, upon acceptance into the plan, and to pay any and all additional fees directly to the providing dentists of the plan. We understand that services under this plan can only be received at participating Dental Maintenance International dental offices.

Member Signature ______________________________ Date _________

Spouse Signature ______________________________ Date _________

I/we do hereby authorize payroll deductions to pay the annual membership fee due Dental Maintenance International for this plan.

Primary Subscriber ______________________________ Date __________

Spouse ______________________________________ Date __________

Rates and Fee Examples

The information packet explains that you have included a copy of the membership fees for the various groups, and an example of the savings to members. This is, of course, a marketing tool and you will have to list the fees of one of your member offices to use it. It is an effective way of encouraging enrollments, but you might find it unnecessary. See Appendix C for the list of discounts and Appendix D for the membership fees.

Provider List

The last item in the information packet is the list of the providers who have agreed to participate. Obviously, if you are offering the plan out of your office only, this will not be necessary. But, remember, we are aiming for credibility. The larger the list, the more impressive your plan will look and the easier it will be to sell. As you sign a new doctor to the plan, it will be worth it to update the list and send an updated version to your clients. Remaining dynamic in their eyes is critical. Make this the last page of the information packet, or a separate insert in your brochure to facilitate that constant updating.

Take notice here of one more reason that discount PPO plans are so much easier to manage than capitation plans. Patients can move freely from one office to another within the system. Eliminating the necessity of keeping one group of patients in one specific office as in capitation plans will eliminate some major headaches.

Operation

You have made a contact with an employer. You have solicited his employees, or the members of a group. Now you must wait for them to send in their applications. When they do, it is time to enter the data in the filing program of your computer. You must enter the individual subscribers in your electronic filing system according to the mandates of the program you have selected. Most filing programs will allow you to send a bill to a particular member without ever leaving that program. You should make sure yours will before you purchase it. Enter the data. When the sign-up period is over, count the number of people who joined, and send a bill.

The bill should be used to further your marketing by thanking them for their participation and reminding them that if they encourage their friends to sign up during the next enrollment period, their own premium could be lower. When they pay, enter it into the program, and have that same program print membership cards for them. You can mail the cards directly or send all of them back to the employer and ask him to distribute them to the employees who have elected membership. The cards should be the small business-size cards that can easily fit in a wallet. They should have your logo printed on them, as well as the names of the primary subscriber and his or her dependents. It might be wise to include some sort of code number (call it a validation number) so that you can access their account in the computer easily, in case it is ever necessary to verify eligibility. You do not have to go to the extent of having plastic cards made unless you can afford it. The information will be kept in the computer, and if it is necessary, you can send replacements out for lost cards rapidly and inexpensively.

You will be left now with only the two basic principles of prepaid health care:

1. Do not over-subscribe
2. Provide the best possible service.

Getting Help

One final note about development, marketing, and operation of a simple discount dental plan. You may find that the burdens of properly administering and marketing the plan yourself are simply more than you can handle. If so, you will need to hire some help.

Office people to stuff envelopes and enter data into the computer are not difficult to find, but a good marketing person might be. Contacting and establishing relations with potential clients is one of the most important aspects of any program. It might be wise to hire a professional to help you. An independent insurance agent with contacts in all phases of business in your area might be invaluable. These people have already contacted many of the groups who could end up being good clients for your dental plan.

They have probably established relationships with many of them and would no doubt enjoy an opportunity to offer another product to them. Hire one of these professionals. Give him a respectable percentage of your membership fees. Give him an additional percentage of renewals. It will be worth it!

If you are unable to find a professional to help, look for assistance in your own backyard. Your provider list can be a valuable source of client referrals. As a matter of fact, some of those same providers can act as salesmen for your program as well. Many have considered doing something besides their daily routine in their spare time. Why not give them a chance to sell your plan for you? You will already have everything in place. Allow them to use your system to their advantage. If a provider knows of a group that is almost exclusively in his area and will probably contribute patients to only his office, why not allow him to run through your company? You have the licensing and paperwork requirements satisfied. You have the computer systems in place. Give the provider a percentage of the membership fee and do the paperwork for him. It will not add that much strain to your system. You might as well benefit from the percentage of the fee you will keep rather than not have the patients or the fee. This will make it a win situation for you and the provider, and it will help to endear your system to him.

Simplicity

Which way to proceed should be obvious now to anyone who has read both the capitation and simple discount plan sections of this book. Capitation is a very difficult and complicated concept. It can be done by anyone, but clearly it would be cost-prohibitive for the small solo practitioner—not impossible, but costly. Larger group practices, multiple facility practices, or several groups who have banded together to form an IPA or other entity to act as sponsor for the plan could perhaps find it lucrative to venture into capitation, but whether it will remain a viable competitor to PPOs and small discount plans which lend themselves so easily to the blossoming self-insurance theory remains questionable. As promised earlier, the small solo practitioner who wants to offer some sort of plan to a busness or some other group in his area should see that he need not be stymied by the complexities of capitation. The simple discount plan is the fast track to accomplishing his goals.

SECTION IV

Topics Relevant to Capitation and PPO-Model Plans

Chapter 12 Reinsurance

The function of the governmental agencies established in each state to regulate the activities of indemnifying insurance companies, health care service corporations, HMOs, and any other alternative payment modalities is to protect the public interest. They require insurance companies and service corporations to maintain large amounts of easily liquefiable assets that can be tapped in the event the entity faces economic difficulties. The purpose is to ensure that when their clients submit claims for reimbursement for health care services, the companies will be able to pay them. To accept payments of premiums for the promise to pay claims and then not to do so, would obviously be fraud.

HMOs and their capitation-formatted relatives provide special challenges since they are not obligated to pay for services in cash but rather to deliver the actual services to their clients. No one has figured out a way to store services for a rainy day. Therefore, regulators have insisted that HMOs and capitation companies borrow a concept from the pure insurance companies called *reinsurance.* Reinsurance is a method of protecting HMOs and capitation plans from rapid and total insolvency by accepting financial responsibility for their debts which extend beyond a certain point. As we have pointed out, it is unlikely that you could obtain licensing for your capitation plan without some sort of reinsurance plan in effect.

The HMO Act of 1973 outlines the basics of the reinsurance concept in one of its first subsections:

> "Each HMO shall . . . assume the full financial risk on a prospective basis for the provision of (services) except that (they) may obtain insurance or make other arrangements for the cost of providing to any member (services) the aggregate value of which exceeds $5,000 in any year . . . and obtain insurance or make other arrangements for not more than 90% of the amount by which its costs for any fiscal year exceed 115% of its income for such fiscal year."

This section establishes the two basic types of reinsurance: *individual* and *aggregate.* The best way to think about reinsurance is as stop-loss insurance, because that is in essence what it is. For example, if an HMO collects $500 a year from an individual in capitation premiums, and that patient requires $7,000 dollars worth of treatments in that same year, it is clear that the HMO will lose money. The federal law requires that the HMO purchase an insurance policy that would go into effect as soon as the patient's bills reach $5,000, and cover the additional $2,000. This individual reinsurance policy would in effect limit (or stop) the HMO's loss from $6,500 to $4,500 for that particular patient.

Aggregate stop-loss insurance works in a similar manner except that it is applied to the overall activities of the HMO or capitation plan. Essentially, the entity, in addition to its individual policy, must carry another policy that will cover 90% of any loss which is more than 15% of its total income. So, if a plan takes in $100,000 in premiums in a year, but incurs costs of $115,000, they must have a plan that would pay 90% of the $15,000 deficit or $13,500. This would result in the plan going only $1,500 in debt, which would make it easier to recover in the next year through cost efficiency and increased capitation premiums.

In addition to individual stop-loss and aggregate stop-loss plans, capitated payment systems can ensure that their clients will indeed receive the treatments they require by contracting with outside providers to provide those services to the clients of the plan in the event that they become insolvent at a later date.

Since premium collections sometimes lag behind treatment expenses, HMOs also purchase reinsurance policies to protect them in the event that they are forced to outlay large amounts of cash for services that seem to bunch up too fast and exceed the cash reserves generated by premium payments which may not yet have been received.

Rates

Reinsurance is generally sold by large life insurance companies, such as North American Life and Casualty. The Blue Cross plans and their affiliates have their own life insurance company called BCS Life Insurance which handles all of their reinsurance policies. The indemnifying insurance companies establish their rates based on a complicated set of guidelines that rely heavily on actuarial statistics. The methods used to calculate rates for reinsurance are even more complex and somewhat guarded. They take into account actuarial statistics, regions of the country, demographics of the population base, experience of the management, history of the company, and a host of other data. The safest advice is to contact one of the large life insurance companies, sit down with a representative of their reinsurance department and outline your needs. Be prepared to adjust your capitation rates to compensate for the premiums you will be charged.

Reinsurance and the PPO

Most states are not regulating PPOs or simple discount plans at this time. In the eyes of the insurance commissioners they do not assume any risk, and therefore, legislation necessary to affect regulation has not been passed. They do not require reinsurance of any kind. Some states have foreseen a problem, however, and have attempted to incorporate some rules designed to avoid it. The problem is one of insolvency on the part of the organizing body. Imagine an independent PPO that solicits membership fees from a group of potential patients for the promise that the PPO or discount plan will be able to supply them with a list of providers who will accept a reduced fee for treatments delivered to plan members. Imagine then that this organization fails to find the providers who will accept their rates, or decides to go out of business altogether. What happens to the membership fees collected? Therein lies the problem. It could happen to a large PPO which is a division of an insurance company or an health service corporation as well. While it is unlikely that they would simply go out of business, it is not so unrealistic to imagine that their provider base might suddenly pull out of the program, or that they might be unable to establish a satisfactory base in the first place. We know that this has happened to the United Dental Network of Denver, and recently Health Alliance Plans of Michigan was challenged by a similar threat from their hospital provider base.

The current philosophy in a state like Michigan is "Let the buyer beware." PPOs are not regulated. If a PPO or a discount plan accepts your membership fee and then suddenly goes out of business, it would be just like your health spa suddenly burning to the ground immediately after you pay your yearly membership fee. The consumer would be faced with only two options: institute conventional civil litigation or forget about it.

Discount Limiting

Some states have chosen to try to prevent the situation mentioned above in a couple of ways. First of all, some have set limits upon how deep a discount an individual plan can offer. That is, they have set a limit on the amount below the standard fee for a given service in a given area, that a discounted fee can be. For example if dental crowns are selling for an average of $300 in a given area, the discount cannot exceed 25% or $75. Therefore, table of allowance rates for a non-percentage plan could not be less than $225. The idea is that if a provider discounts too much, he will go out of business or simply lose interest in the plan, or worse yet, be tempted to cut too many corners in the interest of efficiency. By limiting the amount of the discount that he can charge, his solvency will be more predictable.

Bonds and Insurance Policies

Another way to limit the risk to the consumer is to provide for a surety bond that would become effective in the event the plan is unable to fulfill its obligation. Unfortunately this can be a very difficult bridge to cross. Bonds are issued by large companies like Fireman's Fund, Transamerica, Reliance, Ohio Casualty, or INA. The risk suggested by PPO plans and their discount derivatives is so new that no one has given it much consideration. Surety companies may be reluctant to become involved in issuing a bond for a risk when no state statutes exist which mandate that a bond be obtained.

Bonds are contracts between three entities. If one were issued, it would have the effect of establishing a partnership of sorts between the bond company and the PPO to offer a particular product to the consumers (the third party). Under the conventional thinking, in the event that the plan is unable to fulfill its obligations to the consumers, the bond company would have to. It is possible that a new kind of bond could be written that would not obligate the issuing company to fulfill the obligations of the plan but only to return the membership fee to the consumer. This idea would resemble an insurance policy and indeed might become a commingling of concepts. The future of this type of product is unclear.

In any event, whether you are able to obtain a bond or are able to purchase an insurance policy to help you to convince your prospective clients that they should participate in your plan, it will be necessary for you to provide some extremely detailed financial data on your company and all of the members of your administrative group. In addition, you will have to provide strong contracts between you and your providers, and perhaps even specialized contracts between you and your subscribers.

If you are interested in obtaining a bond, especially in a state where it is required by statute, you should contact a licensed insurance agent who specializes in surety bonds. An agent who is a member of the National Association of Surety Bond Providers (located in Bethesda, MD) will know how to properly process your requests. Sit down with the agent and outline what it is you require, and let him help you decide whether it is a bond or an insurance policy that would help you the most.

Decreasing Value Trust Accounts

There is one more way to handle this particular problem. If a prospective client group raises the question, you might want to try putting the membership fees in escrow with a reputable third party. This third party might be an interest-bearing bank account, a trust company, an attorney, or a title company. At any rate, set up the account with specific instructions to release only one-twelfth of the yearly membership fee to your company for each month that you do indeed have treatment facilities available for the group's members to visit. If for some reason, you go out of business, or your providers drop out of the plan and you are unable to find new ones for a given month, that month's percentage of the fee will be refunded to the group.

If you are dealing with small businesses and small groups, the question may never come up. It is highly likely that no one from the group will ask about your financial future. This is especially true if you are offering small plans to small groups directly out of your office and you adhere to the principles of delivering good services and not oversubscribing. When you attempt to offer the plan to larger groups, and you begin to involve additional providers, someone might wonder what would happen if they gave membership fees to you and then you were unable to provide services for the group. Will you refund the money? If bonding and reinsurance are not possible, you might try this simple remedy of decreasing value trust accounts. Don't, by the way, try using that term with a banker or a trust institution. They may not understand it. Although it has been used in other forms for years, it is an entirely new concept in the field of health care. It could make participation in the plan from the group's standpoint virtually risk free, and limit your risk as well. Since your expenses come in the very beginning of the plan when you have to do the paperwork involved with mailings, computer entries and membership cards, you are only at risk during a time when it is likely that everything will be in place. This assumes, of course, you do not sell plans when you have no providers.

Chapter 13 Miscellany

California's Knox-Keene Law

Many observers have noticed that California has become the spawning ground for a large school of new ideas and concepts which have gradually migrated to other parts of the country. Not surprisingly, many of the concepts involved with prepaid health care have evolved in California as well. It follows then that some confusion would exist with regard to California's law governing the delivery of health care by alternate financing methods.

Many among those considering the development of a prepaid plan have misinterpreted this law. They have been misled into believing that it effectively outlaws prepaid plans in the state of California, and that when the concept spreads to the rest of the country, prepaid dental plans will become a thing of the past. This simply is not true. Passed in 1975, not long after the federal HMO law was adopted, the Knox-Keene law is one of the oldest state statutes developed to regulate prepaid health care. It does not outlaw prepaid plans; rather it establishes the guidelines under which they must be developed and administered.

Stated simply, the state of California asks that any plan wishing to offer prepaid dentistry to consumer groups submit a plan of operation to the state Department of Corporations. If your plan is one modeled after single-service HMOs, like the dental capitation plans, it will have to follow the guidelines established in the Knox-Keene law. It can be done, but it must follow these guides. If, however, your plan is a simple discount plan modeled after the membership-fee-for-reduced-charges concept, it is possible that it would not be regulated very strongly at all.

In reality the Knox-Keene law in California is no different from similar laws in other states. They don't prevent; they merely guide. The reader should view this general pattern, outlined above, as the norm for the development of dental plans. It is definitely the way it is in many states, and no doubt will be the model that other states, which have not yet established legislation in this area, will follow.

Freedom of Choice

An area of controversy in the field of prepaid dentistry concerns the state laws prohibiting insurers from recommending specific providers to their clients. States such as Utah have adopted such legislation, intended to prevent discrimination towards providers. The effectiveness of legislation which merely says that an insurer cannot influence the choice of a particular provider over another is questionable, especially when economic incentives are so much more powerful. It is simple to avoid giving a direct recommendation when pure financial influence will do the job. Obviously single-service HMO plans and closed panel capitation plans come very close to violating these principles and come under scrutiny much more often. Generally, PPOs have been immune to this problem since nothing prevents them from entering into contracts with providers and/or purchasers. The new breed of exclusive provider organizations, of which the discount-for-membership-fee plan is certainly one, may come closer to violation of such laws than conventional PPO plans.

It appears as though this controversy will be solved by a general loosening of the laws by the states. California has already effectively removed the barrier to those who would establish such plans by passing AB 3480 of June 1982. Florida has chosen the same general path with a new amendment to their insurance regulations which provides that ". . . insurers may, by agreement with insureds, limit payments . . . to services secured by insureds from providers charging alternative rates pursuant to contracts with such insurers." Clearly the effect of this wording is to allow economic discrimination of providers and open the door for both open and closed panel PPOs and single-service HMOs.

Dual Choice

Another concern voiced frequently by those considering developing a prepaid dental plan is the federal "dual choice" requirement. Section 1310 of the Federal Public Health Service Act specifies that certain employers are obligated to offer an opportunity to their employees to join a federally qualified HMO in their area, if they offer another form of health care benefit to those employees.

The concern is that if a prepaid company such as Dental Maintenance International approaches a prospective employer client with an opportunity to join its plan, that it may be necessary for that client to then offer a form of conventional coverage to his employees as well. The answer, simply stated, is probably not.

If DMI conducts its business as we have suggested, it is unlikely that the problem will ever come up, for a variety of reasons. First of all, the "certain employers" specified by the act are those who:

1. Were during any calendar year required to pay their employees the minimum wage specified by Section 6 of the Fair Labor Standards Act
2. Employed 25 or more employees during any calendar quarter of that year
3. Offer their employees a health benefit plan
4. Have received a written request from a federally qualified HMO whose service area includes at least 25 of the residences of its employees

If DMI offers its plan to an employer who has less than 25 employees, which may be a good way to start, the rule would not apply. If it offers its plan to an association, individual, or another member group, the rule would not apply. If it offers its plan to an employer who does not offer dental coverage in any other form, the rule would not apply. If the employer is not in the service area of a federally qualified HMO, the rule would not apply. If it is, but the federally qualified HMO does not offer dental coverage as a supplemental benefit, the rule would not apply. Take note: The regulation does not say that if an employer is offered an alternative health care plan by an entrepreneurial group that it must offer conventional insurance as a dual-choice alternative. This has been one of the major points of confusion. It is the other way around if an employer offers conventional coverage; it must also offer the opportunity to join a federally qualified HMO.

IPAs

If DMI is adamant about offering a single-service HMO plan, which is what dental capitation is, and it is adamant about offering its services to an employer who is restricted by the dual-choice mandate, it may still have an option. Obviously, since it is unlikely that a single-service HMO would ever become federally qualified, it would be impossible for DMI to compete unless its organizers were ambitious enough to attempt the formation of a full-service HMO and seek that federal qualification. It would be just as unlikely that an employer would be willing to pay an HMO which offers dental benefits and the premiums of an outside company such as DMI as well. DMI could, however, offer its plan to the HMO in the form of an IPA.

Chapter Two outlined the basics of the IPA format. Those seriously interested in forming an IPA might find valuable information in *Group and IPA HMOs* by Dustin L. Mackie and Douglas K. Decker (Aspen Publications), *The IPA Concept,* published by the Journal of the American Dental Association in March of 1981, and *The Independent Practice Association,* available from the Department of Health Care Delivery Systems of the American Medical Association. In addition, examples of corporate structure as well as several examples of pertinent contracts can be found in the Nichols Cyclopedia of Legal Forms annotated, volume 7A, available in any law library.

Quality Assurance, Peer Review, and Grievances

The laws governing the licensing of a single-service HMO plan or a dental capitation plan usually specify that some sort of quality-assurance procedure be outlined prior to licensing. A method for sampling the need and appropriateness of the treatments rendered will have to be established as will a grievance procedure for enrollees.

Generally this can be accomplished by means of a letter which describes the grievance procedure and outlines how determinations rendered by the procedure will be carried out. Most local dental societies have already established a good basis for this procedure, and the simplest way to fashion yours is to merely copy an existing format. If the local society is not able to assist you, the state licensing board will be able to. They all have grievance and peer review mechanisms, and if you pattern yours after theirs, chances are good that it will be accepted by the insurance offices.

Since PPOs and discount plans are frequently not regulated, grievance procedures are not mandatory. Sometimes though, a functioning review board of some sort could help sell your plan to skeptical potential clients. It may not be necessary to establish a formal structure for this board as long as you have one in place. Perhaps a committee of professionals who could meet to discuss a complaint by a patient would be sufficient. You may want to include a clause in your provider contract which obligates an individual provider to adhere to recommendations offered by this committee in the event of a dispute. Generally speaking, it would be wise to do your best to satisfy the individual patient as well as possible in an attempt to maintain your credibility. If too many complaints are received about a particular practitioner, then perhaps you should consider dropping that provider from your plan. If you are offering a discounted plan directly out of your own office, the entire question is rendered moot. You are subject to the state review procedures and ultimately to civil litigation just as always.

Group Purchases of Supplies and Lab Services

Traditionally in American business, manufacturers do not deal directly with consumers. Some sort of intermediary usually intervenes to play the role of middleman. In most cases the manufacturers of dental equipment do not sell their products directly to dentists. They sell to suppliers and distributors who then distribute the product to the dentists with an additional fee tacked on for their effort. It is no secret that this is the way the game is played. It is possible that the rules could change. It is a question of horsepower. If a single dentist calls a manufacturer and asks to purchase a product, he will find it impossible. He will be told that he must buy it from a distributor. There is no incentive for the manufacturer to sell a small quantity to a particular dentist. If the dentist calls on behalf of one hundred dentists, all seeking to purchase the same thing, it is highly possible that a transaction could occur. It has been done before. The co-op idea is not new. Unfortunately the logistics of distribution and the establishment of some sort of network linking the individual dentists together has made the concept impractical in the past. If you are successful in establishing a network through the development of your plan and its provider network, it may be just as feasible to make some great bulk purchase in order to help cut costs for your dentists. The concept seems even more feasible in light of the changing attitudes and in some cases, changing laws, which have allowed some suppliers to actually own their own dental offices, as is the case in New Jersey and Wisconsin.

If direct purchases of supplies are not feasible, then it may be possible to accomplish the same goals by dealing directly with the suppliers. One large group in Arizona, which owns many dental offices and fulfills a large number of group capitation contracts, has solved the problem in a simple, although not particularly unique fashion. Every year they calculate what supplies they will need for all of their twenty or so offices. Then, when they have compiled a large order of items which can be stored and dispensed slowly (which does, by the way, include most impression materials) they call all of the supply companies and ask for bids. The supplies are stored in a small area in their central office, and when an office needs something, they merely draw against the store. Not only are supplies available to the individual offices much faster than they would be under the traditional system of receiving a supply item only after it has been on "back order" for a while, but they are able to reduce their overall expenses rather dramatically. As we all know, predictably large markups in dental supplies and equipment provide for keen competition between the various suppliers.

The idea of reducing costs through bulk purchases is not new at all to the dental laboratory business. They deal directly with dentists as the norm. Just about any laboratory will be willing to provide services at reduced rates as long as the volume is high enough. The only problem here is logistics. You have to develop a method of distribution of the cases, and a method for establishing who pays for what. You can provide a list to the laboratory of providers in the system who are to receive discounts and then pay a refund after so many cases received, or you can run all of the cases through your central office and perform the discount calculations outside of the laboratory, or you can devise any one of a variety of systems, some of which are already in use. This is clearly another example of how networking of offices can be economically sound and can help your providers offset the discounts they must grant on their services.

Selling the Business

The idea of dental laboratory and even dental supply companies owning dental offices is an interesting one. The state of Wisconsin is making it legal now for entities other than dentists to own dental offices. In New Jersey, dental suppliers are now involved with the ownership of dental offices; they merely hire dentists to perform the services. In Michigan, a large publicly owned dental laboratory has bypassed the rule preventing non-dentists from owning offices by handling all of the financing for a chain of large clinics in one of the regional department stores. While they do not own the offices outright, their financial arrangement with the dentist who does, effectively allows them total control, including the right to replace the dentist at will.

The theory here makes good sense from the lab's point of view. Think of it like a chicken farmer, who traditionally must sell his product only to poultry distributors and must rely on them for his market, but decides one day to open his own Colonel Smith's restaurant so that he can market his product directly to the consumer. The dental laboratory usually sells their crowns, for example, only to dentists—somewhat difficult customers. With this arrangement the lab can direct the activities of the dentist and market their products more directly to the consumer. Not only do they profit from having a captive market in the form of the dentists they employ, they share in the revenue of the dental office as a whole.

Here lies an opportunity for those who have been successful in developing prepaid dental plans. Dental laboratories, which frequently have been able to accumulate more cash than the average dentist, will begin to purchase more and more dental offices as the economic realities of that move become obvious. Soon the labs will seek to control another aspect of the financial equation, whereby money taken out of the pockets of the patients filters through the dental office and ultimately ends up in their accounts. Soon they will seek to control the flow of the money from the patients to the dental office at its source, just as the insurance companies have. A well-developed network dental plan could fit so easily into the picture at this point that you may find it very easy to sell yours to one of these entities and retain a position as consultant. This corollary opportunity riding on the development of one of these programs could be a valuable asset when retirement time comes along.

PPO Ownership

Some question has arisen regarding the ownership of a PPO. Many have wondered whether PPOs should be sponsored by insurance companies or the providers, or the employers paying the bills, or an outside entrepreneur. The answer, of course, is yes in all cases. Any of these entities can and do sponsor PPOs. Insurance companies can do so to decrease the total amount of claims paid while maintaining a constant ratio of profit to premiums received. Providers can sponsor one to help increase patient bases and perhaps even share in profits generated from premiums and membership fees. Employers can establish one to help decrease costs of self-insurance programs. And finally, entrepreneurs can form one as a profit-oriented venture. This is what most of this book has been directed towards, with the dentist acting as both the provider and the entrepreneur.

In some situations, that dual role has been accomplished by a single dentist offering a discount plan out of his office, for his own patients. In others, it has been accomplished by a group of dentists banding together and offering a more comprehensive plan, either directly through hands-on management, or indirectly by stock purchases of a central corporation, such as a formal provider-sponsored PPO, which then handles the management. The point is that providers are operating on both sides of the financial equation, as providers and as business managers, once the so called "third parties." It is this duality of consciousness which may help to return control of the industry to those most closely involved.

APPENDICES

Appendix A

Insurance Commission offices in the U.S.

Alabama
Michael DeBellis
Commissioner of Insurance
135 S. Union St.
Montgomery, AL 36130-3401
(205)269-3550

Alaska
John L. George
Commissioner of Insurance
Pouch D
Juneau, AK 99811
(907)485-2515

Arizona
S. David Childers
Commissioner of Insurance
1601 W. Jefferson
Phoenix, AZ 85034-2217
(602)255-5400

Arkansas
Robert Eubanks III
Commissioner of Insurance
400-18 University Tower Bldg.
Little Rock, AR 72204
(501)371-1325

California
Bruce Bunner
Commissioner of Insurance
600 South Commonwealth Ave.
14th Floor
Los Angeles, CA 90005
(213)736-2551

Colorado
John Kezek
Commissioner of Insurance
303 W. Colfax
5th Floor
Denver, CO 80204
(303)620-4300

Connecticut
Peter W. Gillies
Commissioner of Insurance
165 Capitol Ave.
Room 425, State Office Bldg.
Hartford, CT 06106
(203)566-5275

Delaware
David W. Levinson
Commissioner of Insurance
21, The Green
Dover, DE 19901
(302)736-4251

District Of Columbia
Marguerite C. Stokes
Commissioner of Insurance
614 H St.
North Potomac Building, Suite 512
Washington, D.C. 20001
(202)727-7419

Florida
Bill Gunter
Commissioner of Insurance
State Capitol Plaza Level 2
Tallahassee, FL 32301
(904)488-3440

Georgia
Warren Evans
Commissioner of Insurance
7th Floor West Tower
Floyd Building
2 Martin Luther King Dr.
Atlanta, GA 30334
(404)656-2056

Hawaii
Mario Ramil
Commissioner of Insurance
P.O. Box 3614
Honolulu, HI 96811
(808)548-6522

Idaho
Wayne Soward
Commissioner of Insurance
700 West State St.
Boise, ID 83720
(208)334-2250

Illinois
John E. Washburn
Commissioner of Insurance
320 West Washington
Fourth Floor
Springfield, IL 62767
(217)782-4515

Indiana
Harry E. Eakin
Commissioner of Insurance
509 State Office Building
Indianapolis, IN 46204
(317)232-2386

Iowa
Bruce W. Foudree
Commissioner of Insurance
State Office Building G23
Ground Floor
Des Moines, IA 50319
(515)281-5705

Kansas
Fletcher Bell
Commissioner of Insurance
420 Southwest 9th St.
Topeka, KS 66612
(913)296-3071

Kentucky
Gilbert McCarty
Commissioner of Insurance
239 W. Main St.
P.O. Box 517
Frankfort, KY 40602
(502)564-3630

Louisiana
Sherman A. Bernard
Commissioner of Insurance
P.O. Box 94214
Baton Rouge, LA 70804
(504)342-5238

Maine
Theodore T. Briggs
Commissioner of Insurance
State Office Building
State House, Station #34
Augusta, ME 04333
(207)289-3101

Maryland
Edward J. Muhl
Commissioner of Insurance
501 St. Paul Pl.
7th Floor South
Baltimore, MD 21202
(301)659-6300

Massachusetts
Peter Hiam
Commissioner of Insurance
100 Cambridge St.
Boston, MA 02202
(617)727-3333

Michigan
Herman W. Coleman
P.O. Box 30220
Lansing, MI 48909
(517)373-0220

Minnesota
Michael Hatch
Commissioner of Insurance
500 Metro Square Building
Fifth Floor
St. Paul, MN 55101
(612)296-6848

Mississippi
George Dale
Commissioner of Insurance
1804 Walter Sillers Bldg.
P.O. Box 79
Jackson, MS 39205
(601)359-3569

Missouri
Lewis R. Christ
Commissioner of Insurance
301 E. High St., 6 North
P.O. Box 690
Jefferson City, MO 65102
(314)751-2451

Montana
Andrea Bennett
Commissioner of Insurance
Mitchell Building
P.O. Box 4009
Helena, MT 59604
(406)444-2040

Nebraska
Michael J. Dugan
Commissioner of Insurance
301 Centennial Mall South
State Office Building
P.O. Box 94699
Lincoln, NE 68509
(402)471-2201

Nevada
David Gates
Commissioner of Insurance
Nye Building
201 South Falls St.
Carson City, NV 89710
(702)885-4270

New Hampshire
Louis Bergeron
Commissioner of Insurance
169 Manchester St.
Concord, NH 03301
(603)271-2261

New Jersey
Hazel Frank Gluck
Commissioner of Insurance
201 East State St.
Box CN 325
Trenton, NJ 08625
(609)292-5363

New Mexico
Vincente B. Jasso
Commissioner of Insurance
PERA Building
P.O. Box Drawer 1269
Santa Fe, NM 87504-1269
(505)827-4542

New York
James P. Corcoran
Commissioner of Insurance
160 W. Broadway
New York, NY 10013
(212)602-0429 (in state only)
(800)324-3736 (toll free)
(518)474-6630 (in Albany)

North Carolina
James E. Long
Commissioner of Insurance
Dobbs Building
P.O. Box 26387
Raleigh, NC 27611
(919)733-7343
(800)662-7777 (toll free)

North Dakota
Earl R. Pomeroy
Commissioner of Insurance
Capitol Building
Bismarck, ND 58505
(701)224-2440

Ohio
George Fabe
Commissioner of Insurance
2100 Stella Ct.
Columbus, OH 43215
(614)466-3584

Oklahoma
Gerald Grimes
Commissioner of Insurance
408 Will Rogers Memorial Bldg.
Oklahoma City, OK 73105
(405)521-2828

Oregon
Josephine M. Driscoll
Commissioner of Insurance
158 12th St., N. E.
Salem, OR 97310
(503)378-4271

Pennsylvania
George F. Grode
Acting Commissioner of Insurance
Strawberry Square
13th Floor
Harrisburg, PA 17120
(717)787-5173

Rhode Island
Clifton A. Moore
Commissioner of Insurance
100 North Maine St.
Providence, RI 02903
(401)277-2223

South Carolina
John G. Richards
Commissioner of Insurance
1612 Marion St.
P.O. Box 100105
Columbia, SC 27202-3105
(803)737-6160

South Dakota
Susan L. Walker
Commissioner of Insurance
Insurance Building
320 North Nicolet
Pierre, SD 57501
(605)773-3563

Tennessee
John C. Neff
Commissioner of Insurance
114 State Office Bldg.
Nashville, TN 37219
(615)741-2241

Texas
Doyce R. Lee
Commissioner of Insurance
1110 San Jacinto Blvd.
Austin, TX 78701-1998
(512)463-6169

Utah
Roger C. Day
Commissioner of Insurance
160 E. 300 South
P.O. Box 45803
Salt Lake City, UT 84145
(801)530-6400

Vermont
Thomas P. Menson
Commissioner of Insurance
State Office Building
Montpelier, VT 05602
(802)828-3301

Virginia
James M. Thomson
Commissioner of Insurance
700 Jefferson Bldg.
P.O. Box 1157
Richmond, VA 23209
(804)786-3741

Washington
Dick Marquardt
Commissioner of Insurance
Insurance Building AQ21
Olympia, WA 98504
(206)753-7301

West Virginia
Fred E. Wright
Commissioner of Insurance
2100 Washington St. East
Charleston, WV 25305
(304)348-3354

Wisconsin
Thomas P. Fox
Commissioner of Insurance
123 W. Washington St.
P.O. Box 7873
Madison, WI 53703-7873
(608)266-3585

Wyoming
Monty Laver
Acting Commissioner of Insurance
Herschler Bldg.
122 W. 25th St.
Cheyenne, WY 82002
(307)777-7401

American Samoa
Lyle L. Richmond
Acting Commissioner of Insurance
Office of the Governor
Pago Pago, American Samoa 96797
Written complaints only

Guam
Dave Santos
Commissioner of Insurance
855 W. Marine Dr.
Agana, Guam 96910
Written complaints only

Puerto Rico
Juan Antonio Garcia
Commissioner of Insurance
Old San Juan Station
P.O. Box 3508
San Juan, Puerto Rico 00904
(809)724-6565

Virgin Islands
Julio A. Brady
Commissioner of Insurance
Office of Lieutenant Governor
P.O. Box 450
Charlotte Amalie
St. Thomas, Virgin Islands 00801
(809)774-2991

Appendix B

Co-pay Examples

The fees listed below are examples of capitation plan co-pays. They are in no way representative of current fees in any particular plan. They are included here to demonstrate which fees are frequently associated with co-pays and which are not. Your schedule may differ dramatically.

DESCRIPTION	FEE
00100 Clinical Oral Exam	n/c
00110 Initial Oral Exam	n/c
00120 Periodic Oral Exam	n/c
00130 Emergency Oral Exam	n/c
00210 X-ray Full Mouth	n/c
00212 FM X-ray or Pan X-ray	n/c
00220 X-ray or Pan X-ray	n/c
00212 FM X-ray or Pan X-ray	n/c
00220 X-ray Single	n/c
00230 X-ray Each Additional	n/c
00240 X-ray Intraoral Occl.	n/c
00250 X-ray Extraoral	n/c
00260 X-ray Extraoral Add.	n/c
00270 X-ray Bitewing Pair	n/c
00275 X-ray Bitewing Plus	n/c
00278 Ex. Prophy Fl. Bw. X-ray	n/c
00279 Ex. Prophy Bwx. Fms. and/or Pan.	n/c
00280 X-ray Bitewing Add.	n/c
00330 X-ray Panorex	n/c
00400 Tests & Lab Exam	n/c
00410 Bacterial Cultures	n/c

00420 Caries Sucept. Tests	n/c
00460 Pulp Vitality Tests	n/c
00470 Study Casts	n/c
00490 Misc. Tests & Lab Exam	n/c
00920 Consultation Appt.	n/c

PREVENTIVE

01110 Dent. Prophy (Adult)	n/c
01115 Scaling & Curettage	n/c
01120 Dental Prophy (Child)	n/c
01210 Appl. Sodium Fluoride	n/c
01220 Stannous Fluoride	n/c
01225 Fluoride Treatment	n/c
01230 App. Acid Fluoride	n/c
01300 Other Preventive Service	n/c
01310 Dietary Planning	n/c
01330 Home Care Instruction	n/c
01340 Preventative Home Care	n/c
01510 Space Maint (Fixed)	lab
01511 Space Maintainer	lab
01515 Space Maintainer (Stainless)	lab
01520 Space Maint. (Fixed Cast.)	lab
01530 Space Maint. (Rem. Acrylic)	lab
01540 Add. Cla. & Activ. Wire	lab

RESTORATIVE

02110 Amalgam (1 Surf. Decid.)	n/c
02120 Amalgam (2 Surf. Decid.)	n/c
02130 Amalgam (3 Surf. Decid.)	n/c
02131 Amalgam (4 Surf. Decid.)	n/c
02140 Amalgam (1 Surf. Perm.)	n/c
02150 Amalgam (2 Surf. Perm.)	n/c
02160 Amalgam (3 Surf. Perm.)	n/c

02161 Amalgam (4 Surf. Perm.)	n/c
02170 Reinf. Pin Amalgam	n/c
02195 Reinf. Per Pin	n/c
02200 Silicate Restoration	n/c
02210 Silicate Filling	n/c
02300 Acrylic or Plast. Rest.	n/c
02310 Resin 1 Surface	n/c
02320 Resin 2 Surfaces	n/c
02330 1 Surf. Comp. Filling	n/c
02331 2 Surf. Comp. Filling	n/c
02332 3 Surf. Comp. Filling	n/c
02340 Acid Etch Composite	35.00
02370 Pin Attachment Resin	n/c
02500 Inlay Restoration	91.50
02510 Inlay 1 Surface	91.50
02520 Inlay 2 Surfaces	91.50
02530 Inlay 3 Surfaces	91.50
02540 Onlay	112.75
02610 Inlay Porcelain	122.75
02710 Plastic Crown Resin Ven.	124.50
02720 Full Crown Resin Ven.	124.50
02740 Porcelain Crown	158.25
02750 Porcelain W/Metal Crown	148.25
02790 Full Crown	124.50
02810 3/4 Crown	124.50
02830 Stainless Crown	n/c
02840 Temporary Crown	29.50
02841 Composite Core	35.00
02850 Post Core Reinforce	35.00
02890 Crown W/Pin Ext. Tooth	37.50
02891 Crown W/Post Ext. Tooth	n/c
02910 Recement Inlay	n/c
02920 Recement Crown	n/c

02930 Sedative Base	n/c
02940 Sedative Fillings	n/c

ENDODONTICS

03100 Pulp Capping	n/c
03110 Pulp Cap Direct	n/c
03120 Pulp Cap Indirect	n/c
03130 Recalcification	26.25
03200 Pulpotomy	15.50
03210 Therap. Apical Clos.	38.50
03220 Vital Pulpotomy	15.50
03310 RCT 1 Canal	99.75
03320 RCT 2 Canals	120.75
03330 RCT 3 Canals	170.25
03340 RCT 4 Canals	178.50
03420 Apicoectomy W/Retrograde Fill	99.75
03440 Apical Curettage	61.00
03450 Root Amputation	72.50
03910 Ging. Cur. for Endo Reasons Only	n/c
03920 Hemisection	72.50
03990 Emer. Proced. Endo.	n/c

PERIODONTICS

04100 Non. Surg. Serv. Perio.	n/c
04120 Gingival Curettage/Quad	56.75
04210 Gingivoplasty/Quad	56.75
04310 Perio. Care Plaque	33.75
04320 Provis Splint Intra/Per Tooth	22.25
04321 Provis Splint Extra	91.50
04330 Occl. Adjust. Limit	27.50
04331 Occl. Adjust. Complete	56.75
04340 Perio. Sc/Root Pl. Comp.	114.50
04341 Perio. Sc/Root Pl. Part.	33.75

04350 Tooth Move Perio.	n/c
04360 Spc. Perio Apl.	n/c
04600 Gingivectomy/Quad	217.50
04700 Perio. or Osseous Surg. Flap/Quad	251.00

REMOVABLE PROSTHODONTICS

05110 Comp. Upper Dentures	175.25
05120 Comp. Lower Dentures	175.25
05130 Immed. Upper Dentures	185.25
05140 Immed. Lower Dentures	185.25
05210 Flipper Part. No. Cl.	70.25
95215 Temp. Partial Acrylic	70.25
05224 Up Part W/2 Chrome Cl & Rst Acr Base	225.50
05225 Low Par W/2 Chrome Cl & Rst Acr Base	225.50
05231 Low Par 2CL 2 & Rst W/Lin Bar Acr Base	225.50
05241 Low Par 2Cl 2 Rs W/Lin Bar Cast Base	225.50
05251 Up Par W/Crm Cast Fwrk & 2 Cl Acr Base	225.50
05261 Up Par W/Crm Cast Fwrk & 2 Cl Cst Base	225.50
05281 Remove. Unil. Part. Dent.	99.75
05290 Upper Full Cast Partial	235.00
05291 Lower Full Cast Partial	235.00
05400 Adjust Denture	n/c
05410 Adjustment Comp. Dent.	n/c
05420 Adjustment Part. Dent.	n/c
05600 Repairs to Dentures	lab
05615 Rep. Partial Dentures	lab
05630 Replace Additional Teeth	lab
05640 Replace Tooth	lab
05650 Additional Tooth Denture	lab
05660 Additional Tooth Part. Denture	lab
05670 Reatt. Damaged Cl. Denture	lab
05680 Replace Broken Cl. Denture	lab
05690 Additional Clasp With Rest.	lab

05710 Dup. Denture Com.	lab
05720 Dup. Part. Dentures	lab
05730 Reline Denture/Office	25.25
05740 Reline Partial Denture/Office	25.25
05750 Reline Complete Denture/Lab	55.25
05760 Reline Partial Denture/Lab	55.25
05850 Tissue Conditioning	25.25
05115 Upper Economy Denture	95.50
05125 Lower Economy Denture	95.50

FIXED PROSTHODONTICS

06210 Cast Pontic	130.25
06220 Steele's Facing Pontic	128.25
06225 Steele's or Tru-Pontic	128.25
06230 Tru-Pontic Bridges/Per Unit	128.25
06240 Porcelain Metal Pontic	135.25
06250 Resin Veneer Pontic	114.50
06610 Replace Broken Pin Facing	lab
06620 Replace Broken Face Steel	lab
06630 Replace Broken Face & Post 5	lab
06640 Replace Broken Face Acrylic	lab
06650 Replace Broken Tru-Pontic	lab
06660 Repair Recement Face	n/c
06710 Plastic (Acrylic) Crown Abut.	99.75
06720 Resin on Metal Crown	114.50
06750 Porcelain Metal Abut.	135.25
06780 3/4 Metal Abut.	125.50
06790 Full Metal Abut.	125.50
06930 Recement Bridge	n/c
06940 Stress Breaker	lab
06950 Precision Attachment	97.25
06955 Post for Crown (Metal)	35.50
06960 Dowel Pin Metal Crown	30.50

ORAL SURGERY

07100 Simple Extractions	n/c
07110 Routine Extraction	n/c
07120 Routine Ext. Each Add. Tooth	n/c
07200 Surgical Extractions	29.25
07210 Surgical Ext. Erupted	29.25
07220 Soft Tissue Impaction	59.75
07230 Part. Bony Impaction	79.75
07240 Comp. Bony Impaction	105.75
07250 Root Recovery	69.75
07270 Tooth Replantation	29.25
07280 Sur. Exposure Tooth	49.25
07300 Alveoloplasty/Quad	69.25
07510 Incis. Drain Absc.	39.75
07910 Simple Suture	n/c
07940 Ostioplasty/Quad	135.25
07950 Ostio or Perio Graft/Quad	105.00
07960 Frenulectomy	29.25
07970 Exc-Hyper Tissue/Quad	49.25

OTHER SERVICES

09110 Emer. Palliative Treatment	n/c
09230 Nitrous Oxide Anal.	n/c
09310 Consultation	n/c
09430 Office Visit No Treatment	n/c
09440 Office Visit After Hours	n/c
09940 Occl. Adj. Ltd.	29.50
09988 Missed Appointment	7.50

This schedule assumes the use of non-precious metals only. If the enrollee selects gold, there will be an additional charge according to gold's current market value.

Appendix C

Fee Schedule for Discount PPO Plan

SERVICE	MEMBER ALLOWANCE
PREVENTION AND DIAGNOSIS	
Initial Oral Exam	100%
Periodic Oral Exam	100%
Emergency Office Call	100%
Regular Office Call	100%
Consultations	100%
Emergency Palliative Treatment	100%
Study Models	100%
Pulp Vitality Tests	100%
Panoramic X-ray	75%
Bitewing X-rays (4)	75%
X-rays any other type (each)	100%
Cleanings (Adult)	25%
Cleanings (Child)	25%
Fluoride Treatments	75%
Space Maintainers (fxd. unilat.)	60%
FILLINGS OR FOUNDATIONS	
Fillings (Silver, 2 surface)	30%
Fillings (White, 2 surface)	25%
Incisal Edge Filling	25%
Restoration With Pin	100% of pin
Pin Core (Any Material)	35%

Post Core (Cast)	35%
Post Core (Preformed)	40%

CAPS OR CROWNS

Temporary Crown (Plastic)	50%
Stainless Steel Crown	35%
Inlays and Onlays	25%
Full Crowns (Gold)	25%
Full Crowns (Nonprecious)	25%
Porcelain to Metal	25%
All Porcelain Crowns	25%
Recement Crowns or Inlays	100%
Recement Temporaries	100%
Sedative Fillings	100%

ROOT TREATMENTS

Pulp Capping (Direct or Indirect)	100%
Pulpotomy	25%
Apical Closure	20%
Root Canal (One Canal)	35%
Root Canal (Two Canals)	20%
Root Canal (Three or More Canals)	20%
Apicoectomy	25%
Apical Curretage	40%
Retro Amal	20%
Hemisection	40%
Emergency Endodontic Procedure	50%

GUM TREATMENTS

Occlusal Adjustments (Simple)	100%
Occlusal Adjustments	50%
Gingival Curretage (Full Mouth)	25%
Root Planning and Curretage	25%

Gingivoplasty (Quad)	25%
Gingivectomy (Quad)	25%
Splinting	25%
Flap Surgery, Osseous (Sextant)	25%
Specialized Full Perio Case	25%

ORAL SURGERY

Simple Extraction	40%
Additional Tooth	40%
Surgical Extraction (Erupted)	35%
Soft Tissue Impaction	25%
Partial Bony Impaction	25%
Complete Bony Impaction or Diff.	20%
Root Recovery	25%
Tooth Replantation W/Stab.	25%
Surgical Exposure	25%
Alveoloplasty (Quad)	35%
Biopsy	20%
Incision and Drain (Simple)	50%
Incision and Drain (Complex)	20%
Simple Suture	50%
Ostioplasty (Quad)	20%
Frenulectomy	20%
Exc Hyperplastic Tissue (Quad)	20%

PROSTHODONTICS

Complete Dentures (Upper or Lower)	20%
Immediate Dentures (Upper or Lower)	20%
Flippers	25%
Partials (Upper)	25%
Partials (Lower)	25%
Reline (Office)	25%
Reline (Laboratory)	25%

Tissue Conditioning	35%
Replace Tooth on Denture	35%
Repair Acrylic (Simple)	50%
Repair Acrylic (Complex)	35%
Other Repairs (Add Teeth & Clasp)	25%
Fixed Bridges	25%
Recement Bridges	100%

COSMETIC DENTISTRY (Not covered by most other plans)

Bonding & Veneers	25%

Appendix D

Membership Fees for Discount Plans

DENTAL MAINTENANCE INTERNATIONAL

Membership Rates

CLASSIFICATIONS	YEARLY MEMBERSHIP
NON-GROUP	
INDIVIDUALS	
Adult	76.00
Child	59.00
FAMILIES	
2 Members	135.00
3 Members	192.00
4 Members	240.00
5 Members	284.00
6 or more	325.85
GROUP	
# OF PRIMARY SUBSCRIBERS: 2–5	
INDIVIDUALS	
Adult	74.00
Child	57.00
FAMILIES	
2 Members	132.00
3 Members	189.00
4 Members	233.70

5 Members	276.00
6 or more	316.35

 # OF PRIMARY SUBSCRIBERS: 6–10

INDIVIDUALS	
Adult	72.00
Child	55.00
FAMILIES	
2 Members	128.50
3 Members	183.50
4 Members	226.00
5 Members	267.00
6 or more	306.00

 # OF PRIMARY SUBSCRIBERS: 11–20

INDIVIDUALS	
Adult	70.00
Child	52.00
FAMILIES	
2 Members	125.50
3 Members	177.50
4 Members	217.55
5 Members	256.00
6 or more	292.50

 # OF PRIMARY SUBSCRIBERS: 21–50

INDIVIDUALS	
Adult	68.00
Child	50.00
FAMILIES	
2 Members	121.50
3 Members	171.50

4 Members	211.00
5 Members	248.00
6 or more	281.00

 # OF PRIMARY SUBSCRIBERS: 51–100

INDIVIDUALS	
Adult	66.00
Child	48.50
FAMILIES	
2 Members	118.00
3 Members	166.50
4 Members	205.00
5 Members	240.50
6 or more	273.00

 # OF PRIMARY SUBSCRIBERS: 100–500

INDIVIDUALS	
Adult	64.00
Child	47.00
FAMILIES	
2 Members	114.50
3 Members	161.00
4 Members	199.00
5 Members	233.00
6 or more	265.00

 # OF PRIMARY SUBSCRIBERS: 500–1000

INDIVIDUALS	
Adult	62.00
Child	45.50
FAMILIES	
2 Members	111.00

3 Members	156.50
4 Members	193.00
5 Members	226.00
6 or more	257.00

 # OF PRIMARY SUBSCRIBERS: 1000 OR MORE

INDIVIDUALS	
Adult	60.00
Child	44.00
FAMILIES	
2 Members	107.50
3 Members	151.50
4 Members	187.00
5 Members	220.00
6 or more	250.00

Appendix E

For Further Reading

"There Are Quality Prepaid Dental Plans." *Dental Economics* (August 1988).

"Making Sense Out of Capitation." *Dental Economics* (February 1988).

"Massachusetts Plan Annoys Excluded Dentists." *Dentist* (January 1988).

Alternate Delivery Systems. Aspen, 1987.

"How to Evaluate Capitation Plans." *Dental Economics* (June 1987).

"In-Office Dental Plan Boosts Solo Practice." *Dental Economics* (June 1987).

"Dentists Form Alternatives to Closed-Panel Capitation." *Dentist* (May 1987).

"Direct Pay: Abuse Risk?" *Future Dentistry* (May 1987).

"Insurance Expert Discusses Options." *Dentistry Today* (May 1987).

"Plans and Scams." *ADA News* (May 1987).

"Capitation Contracts: Provider Beware." *Dental Management* (April 1987).

"Direct Reimbursement Patrons Forge Ahead." *Dentistry* (April 1987).

"Study Finds HMOs Don't Reduce Costs." *The Detroit News* (April 3, 1987).

"Capitation Group Hunts Down Facts." *Dentist* (March 1987).

"ADA Eyes Study on Capitation." *ADA News* (January 1987).

HMO PPO Directory. Whole World Books, 1986.

Policies on Dental Care Programs. ADA Council on Dental Care Programs, 1986.

The PPO Debate. ADA Council on Dental Care Programs, 1986.

"Dentists Dodging Popular PPOs." *Dentistry Today* (December 1986).

"Before You Join: How to Evaluate a Dental Capitation Program." *Dental Management* (October 1986).

"HMOs Drawing Fire from Protest Groups." *ADA News* (October 1986).

"Misconceptions About Capitation." *Dental Economics* (October 1986).

"Beware the Pitfalls of Provider Contracts." *Dental Economics* (September 1986).

"Capitation on the Rise: Insurance Companies are Climbing Aboard." *Dental Economics* (July 1986).

"FTC Prepares PPO Study." Parts 1, 2. *Dentist* (July, August 1986).

"Coming to Terms with Prepaid Dentistry." *Dental Economics* (July 1986).

"Caution on Capitation Practice." *Journal of the Southern California Dental Association* (June 1986).

"Capitation: Can It Be a Viable Part of Your Practice?" Parts 1, 2. *Journal of the Indiana Dental Association* (May, June 1986).

Evaluating the Performance of the Prepaid Medical Group: A Management Audit Manual. CTR Res. Ambulatory, 1985.

Management Accounting for Fee-For-Service Prepaid Medical Group. CTR Res. Ambulatory, 1985.

The New Health Care Market: A Guide to PPOs for Purchasers, Payors, and Providers. Dow Jones-Irwin, 1985.

The PPO Handbook. Aspen, 1985.

"Health Care Containment: What the Corporations Want." *Journal of Dental Administration Practice* 2 (1985).

"The PPO Debate: An Alphabet Soup." *Journal of Dental Practice Administration* 2 (April/June 1985).

"The Alphabet Soup: More on the Debate." *Journal of Dental Practice Administration* 2 (July/September 1985).

"Direct Reimbursement Dental Benefit Plans Require Aggressive Marketing." *Dental Economics* (November 1985).

"Are PPOs Really Bringing in More Patients?" *Dental Management* (October 1985).

"Capitation Dentistry: Can It Work for You?" *Journal of Dental Practice Administration* (October/December 1985).

"Structuring Prepaid Dental Plans to Accomodate Consumer Tastes and Preferences." Parts 1, 2. *Dental Assistant* (September, October 1985).

"California Delta Takes Capitation Plan Management." *American Dental Association News* April 15, 1985.

"Direct Reimbursement: Eliminating the Middlemen." *Dental Economics* (April 1985).

Attorneys and Physicians Examine PPOs. National Health Lawyers Association, 1984.

Frost and Sullivan. *HMO Marketplace.* 1984. (Order #A1371 from the Knowledge Index, a computer database network).

Preferred Provider Organizations. National Health Lawyers Association, 1984.

Preferred Provider Organizations and Alternative Health Care Delivery Systems. Pennsylvania Bar Institute, 1984.

Cohen. *Preferred Provider Organizations: Planning, Structure, and Operation.* Aspen, 1984.

"Alternate Dental Delivery Systems and Reimbursement Mechanisms." *Detroit Dental Bulletin, Supplement* (1984).

State Regulations of Preferred Provider Organizations: A Survey of State Statutes. American Hospital Association, 1984.

"What's the Future of Fee-For-Service Dentistry?" *Dental Management* (September 1984).

"Denver-Based UDN Goes Bankrupt." *American Dental Association News* August 27, 1984.

"Chicago Dental Clinic Franchise Contracts for Service/Supplies. Patterson and J. Morita. *Proofs,* May 1984.

"The PPO Dilemma: Questions to a Network President." *Dental Economics* (April 1984).

"What to Look for in a Dental PPO." *Dental Economics* (April 1984).

"PPOs: An Executive's Guide." *Pluribus Press* (January 1984).

Actuarial Issues in the Fee-For-Service Prepaid Medical Group. CTR Res. Ambulatory, 1983.

Alternative Benefit Plan Models: A Comparison of Contractual Arrangements. Council on Dental Care Programs of the ADA, 1983.

Chairman's letter to colleagues. Dental Care Programs of the ADA, 1983.

Management Information Systems for the Fee-For-Service Prepaid Medical Group. CTR Res. Ambulatory, 1983.

Minutes of Annual Dental Prepayment Conference. Council of Dental Care Programs, 1983.

PPOs and Dentistry. Council on Dental Care Programs, 1983.

The Role of the Medical Director in the Fee-for-Service Prepaid Medical Group. CTR Res. Ambulatory, 1983.

"The Payoff in Prepaid Dentistry." *Dental Management* (November 1983).

"Interstudy Researchers Trace Progress of PPOs, Provide Insight into Future Growth." *FAH Review* (July/August 1983).

"Preferred Provider Organizations and Dentistry." *Journal of the American Dental Association* (July 1983).

"Evaluating Capitation Finances in a Dental Practice." *General Dentistry* (April 1983).

Legal Issues in the Fee-For-Service Prepaid Medical Group. CTR Res. Ambulatory, 1982.

Legal forms for HMO contracts. *Nichols Cyclopedia.* Vol 7A, 1982.

"Competition: Getting a Fix on PPOs." *Hospitals* (November 1982).

"Alternative Dental Systems: Four Experts Examine Their Impact." *Journal of the American Dental Association* (October 1982).

"The Delivery of Dental Care: An Assessment of Five Alternate Systems." *Journal of the American Dental Association* (September 1982).

"Capitation: Curse or Cure?" *Dental Economics* (June 1982).

"Competitive Markets Spawning PPOs." *American Medical News* (May 1982).

"We Can't Be Passive About Capitation." *Dental Economics* (February 1982).

"Move Over HMOs, Make Room for PPOs." *Perspective* (Winter 1982).

Group and IPA HMOs. Aspen, 1981.

The Source Book of Health Insurance Data. U.S. Dept. of Health, 1981 and 1980.

Understanding Dental Prepayment. American Dental Association, 1981.

"A Brief Look at Non-Traditional Dental Practices." *Dental Economics* (November 1981).

"An Alternative Dental Delivery System." Parts 1, 2. *General Dentistry* (September, October 1981).

"Capitation: Some Truths and Myths." *Journal of the American Dental Association* (July 1981).

"Prepay Dentistry Can Work for You." *Dental Management* (July 1981).

"Capitation Dental Plans: A New Slant." *Journal of the Michigan Dental Association* (June 1981).

"Capitation Dental Programs." *Journal of the Michigan Dental Association* (June 1981).

"Capitation: One Dentist's Experience." *Journal of the Michigan Dental Association* (June 1981).

"Group Prepaid Dental Plans: How They'll Change the Way You Practice." *New Dentist* (April 1981).

"The IPA Concept: Its Implications for Dentistry." *Journal of the American Dental Association* (March 1981).

"Capitation Clinics Close Doors." *Dental Economics* (February 1981).

"The Closed Panel That Failed." *Dental Survey* (January 1981).

HMOs and the Politics of Health System Reform. American Hospital Association, 1980.

The Individual Practice Association. The American Medical Association, 1980.

Skills Development for the HMO Managers of the 1980's. Group Health Association of America, 1980.

"Network Capitation Practices: A New Concept." *Community Dental Oral Epidemiology* 8 (1980): 351–354.

"Understanding Capitation." Parts 1, 2, 3, 4. *Journal of the Michigan Dental Association* (December 1980, January, February, March 1981).

"Heiser's Capitation Empire Expands." Parts 1, 2. *Dental Economics* (September, October 1980).

"Coordination of Benefits in Dental Prepayment Programs." *Journal of the American Dental Association* (September 1980).

"Understanding Capitation Dentistry." *Journal of the Kentucky Dental Association* (July 1980).

"Prepaid Group Practice." *The New Dentist* 11 (1980): 27.

Health Maintenance Organization Dental Delivery System. U.S. Department of Health, Education and Welfare, 1979.

HMO Quality Assurance Compliance. Group Health Association of America, 1979.

Management and Policy Issues in HMO Development. Group Health Association of America, 1979.

Statement on Dental Prepayment. ADA Council on Dental Programs, 1979.

"Capitation: A Comparison of Delivery Systems." *Journal of the Southern California Dental Association* (September 1979).

"Controlling the Cost of Dental Care." *American Journal of Public Health* (July 1979).

"The Dental Entrepreneurs." *Dental Management* (June 1979).

"Denture Service Use in a Selected Prepaid Dental Program." *Journal of the American Dental Association* (July 1979).

"Prepaid Dental Care: Patterns of Use and Sources of Premiums." American Journal of Public Health (July 1979).

"Capitation: Is It a Threat?" *Dental Economics* (March 1979).

Proceedings of the Conference on Dental Prepayment. ADA Council on Dental Care Programs, 1978.

"The Inclusion of Capitation Reimbursement in the Solo Practice." *Journal of Public Health Dentistry* (Spring 1978).

"Is a Capitation System for Children's Dentistry Practicable?" *Lancet* (July 1977).

"Results of the Minnesota Dental Association Prepaid Dental Care Survey." Parts 1, 2. *Journal of the Northwest Dental Association* (March, April 1977).

"Capitation Dentistry: A Quasi-Experimental Evaluation." *Medical Care* (March 1977).

The HMO Model and Its Application. VCH Publishers, 1976.

"Where Should Prepaid Dental Care Be Going?" *Journal of the Oregon Dental Association* (December 1976)

"Prepaid Dental Insurance: Direct Payment Not Likely in Near Future." *Journal of the National Association of Dental Laboratories* (March 1976).

"A Viewpoint of Anesthesia in Dentistry and its Relation to Prepaid Dental Plans." *Journal of the Macomb Dental Association* (February 1976).

The Design of a Health Maintenance Organization: A Handbook for Practitioners. Praeger Publishers, 1975.

HMO Handbook. Aspen, 1975.

"Prepaid Dental Plans." *Journal of the Ontario Dental Society* (October 1975).

"Dentistry Responds to the Demand for Change." *Journal of the Michigan Dental Association* (June 1975).

Prepaid Dental Care Technical Assistance Manual. Jerold Enterprises, 1974.

"Standards for Dental Prepayment Programs." *American Dental Association Leadership Bulletin* (December 1974).

"California Dental Service: Pacesetter for Prepayment." *Journal of the American Dental Organization* (October 1974).

"The Growth and Growing Pains of Dental Prepayment." *Journal of the American Dental Association* (October 1974).

"Health Maintenance Organizations: A Federal Protege." *Journal of the American Dental Association* (October 1974).

"Dental Experience in the Prepaid Group Practice." *Journal of the New Jersey Dental Association* (Spring 1974).

"Methodology of Capitation Payment to Group Dental Practice and Effects of Such Payment on Care." *Health Services Reports* (January/February 1974).

Title 42 of the Public Health and Welfare Act, Subchapter 11, 1973.

"Observation of Selected Dental Services Under Two Prepayment Mechanisms." *American Journal of Public Health* (August 1973).

"Prepaid Dental Health Care Systems." *Journal of the Missouri Dental Society* (March 1972).

"Closed Panels and Capitation: What Do They Mean?" *Journal of the Southern California Dental Association* (February 1972).

"Prepaid Dental Plan for Ford UAW Workers." *Journal of the American Dental Association* (February 1972).

"Private Group Practice Utilizing Capitation Prepayment." *Journal of Kentucky Medical Association* (January 1972).

"Peer Review and Prepaid Dental Insurance." *Bulletin of the San Fernando Dental Society* (January, June 1972).

An Experiment in Dental Prepayment: The Naismith Dental Plan. U.S. Department of Health, 1970.

"Delta Dental Plans Association Prepaid Dental Care Coverage: The Need to Prove It's Different." *Journal of the American Dental Association* (June 1970).

"Prepaid Dental Care and the Dental Assistant." *Dental Assistant* (February 1970).

Proceedings of a Workshop on the Place of Periodontics in Prepaid Health Care Plans. American Academy of Periodontology and the Health Insurance Council, April 1969.

Prepaid Dentistry: A Case Study. Center for Labor Research and Education, University of California, 1967.

Proceedings of Workshop on Principle of Prepaid Dental Care. Metropolitan District Dental Society, Boston, 1964.

Dental Care in a Group Purchase Plan. U.S. Department of Health, 1959.

Cost Controls for Health Benefits—How the HMO Does It. Towers Perrin Forster & Crosby discussion paper.

The Dental Service Corporation in a Public Assistance Program. U.S. Dept. of Health and Welfare.

HMO—An Alternative to Traditional Health Insurance. Insurance Consumer Alert. Insurance Bureau, Michigan Dept. of Licensing.

A Practical Guide to Physician-sponsored HMO Development. American Soc. Internal Medicine.

Speaking of Prepaid Dental Care. U.S. Dept. of Health, Education, and Welfare.

INDEX

Index

A

B

C

D

G

H

I

J

K

L

N

O

P

Q

R

S

T

U

V

W